The Truth About 'ME'

"It's not Rocket science. It's Neuroscience"

Catherine Vandome

© Catherine Vandome

Published in 2024 by The Bruges Group

ISBN: 978-1-7390920-8-5

Front cover photograph taken by Sarah Flanagan

The Bruges Group Publications Office
246 Linen Hall, 162-168 Regent Street, London W1B 5TB
www.brugesgroup.com

Bruges Group publications are not intended to represent a corporate view of European and international developments. Contributions are chosen on the basis of their intellectual rigour, and their ability to open up new avenues for debate.

Scan me for Bruges Group

Twitter ✖ @brugesgroup, LinkedIn 🔗 @brugesgroup
GETTR 🔵 @brugesgroup, Telegram ✈ t.me/brugesgroup, Facebook 🅕 @brugesgroup
Instagram 🔴 @brugesgroup, YouTube 🔴 @brugesgroup

This is the story of the Actress, the Osteopath, and the Minister of Defence. Not to be confused with the 1963 Profumo affair, which led to the 1989 movie Scandal. However, the scandal here is that it took over a hundred years to correctly diagnose the health condition 'Myalgic Encephalomyelitis' (ME) as a physical condition, and not a psychological one.

"Please welcome onto the stage...Miss Cathy Vandome!"

The enthusiastic ripple of the audience's applause resonates through the auditorium and this is my cue to enter from down stage left. Inhaling sharply, I clench my stomach tightly, fully aware that my outfit is leaving very little to the imagination. Smoothing down the fabric of my jet-black leotard, sheen hot pants and shimmer tights, I readjust my tightly pinned black fringe cropped wig. All the time I am trying not to smudge my newly applied bright red gloss lipstick. I balance precariously in the wings in six-inch silver sequinned heels, and take in the unparalleled feeling of the excitement of performing live on stage.

The applause begins to fade as the musical introduction fires up. Adrenaline surges through my veins and I momentarily stop breathing. A bead of sweat from the heat of the multi-coloured bright stage lights escapes my wig and travels slowly down the left side of my cheek. My eyes are wide open in a theatrical combination of sheer pleasure and sheer fear, my breathing laboured, as I continue to hold in my stomach, in an attempt to defy gravity. My throat is now so dry I can barely swallow. I am suddenly aware of how important this show is. To be invited to perform in my own hometown on the Charter Theatre stage in Preston, for The Preston Guild Gig 2012 Celebrations, with billings including; 'The Ronnie Scott's Jazz Orchestra', Stand-up Comedian Phil Cool, and Headline Singer and Musician Tony Christie.

From backstage I begin my opening number, hoping that my microphone is not picking up the thumping sound of my heart beating right out of my chest. I become blissfully alive as I transition into character. I feel exhilarated! This is it. This intoxication is what I live for. This is what drives and excites me. The stage is my whole world, there is no greater feeling than this…

Contents

List of Illustrations

FOREWORD
by Stand-up Comedian Patrick Monahan.

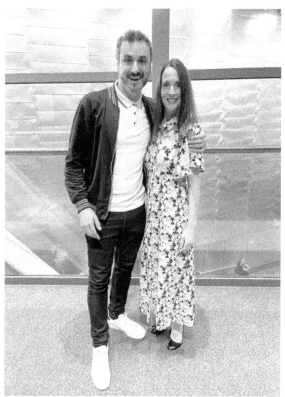

Catherine Vandome with Stand-up Comedian Patrick Monahan.

Me and my mate Catherine Vandome met in 2001. I have known Catherine (or Cathy as I know her), since I first started doing stand-up comedy back in 1911. The Comedy and Cabaret circuit back then was spit and saw dust, with lots of small venues with as many stains on the carpets as there were audience members. Some gigs might have only had about five or six people watching, including Charlie Chaplin (or someone who had a moustache and looked like Charlie Chaplin).

I remember Cathy, like me, was always so upbeat about doing the show, we loved performing in front of any audience, whether they wanted to be there or not. Sometimes they wanted the shows to go on for longer even though we didn't have any more material to perform.

Cathy was lucky, as well as doing stand-up, stories and routines, she had and still has, an amazing singing voice, so she could break out into impressions and songs at the drop of a hat. It was always easy for Cathy to do an encore.

I couldn't sing or dance. If I wanted the audience to stay longer once my material had run out, I would simply lock the doors and just keep talking at them, until the police arrived or Cathy helped wave me off stage and let the audience members out of the fire exit, before I could get to my scribbled stand-up notes and try some new stand-up material on them.

Cathy, like me, had ventured from the North of England, she from the glamorous Northwest and I from the unruly Northeast, down to the big smoke of London. We were two northerners from towns that had never seen so much excitement and so many people before.

I remember backstage at the gigs. We'd stare at the audience coming in to take their seats. As there were no proper backstage or green rooms at some of these early gigs, it was just chairs at the back of a small room behind the few chairs that were set out for the audience.

Cathy and I used to chat and observe the audience coming in, hearing all their different accents and languages. Many of the audiences were from Europe or farther overseas, and English wasn't their first language. In fact, some of the audience couldn't speak English at all. This really worried some of the other acts who were about to perform, but it didn't worry Cathy or I because we both lived in towns in the north of England that can't speak proper English and THESE people ARE English! Cathy then went on to do amazing performances overseas, performances as a great 'Jessie J'. I remember thinking that I wished I could sing. Cathy just said to me, "You could if you tried". I obviously couldn't, but Cathy was always so positive and she made everyone she met feel like Orville and Keith Harris. Every time I said, "I can't" Cathy would simply reply, "You can!"

I've known Cathy for over eighty years and here's to another eighty years of friendship and show business.

Patrick Monahan – Stand-up Comedian. Winner of ITV1 Stand-up comedy 'Show me the funny' hosted by Jason Manford at the London Hammersmith Apollo in 2011. TV credits include BBC1, BBC2, ITV1, ITV2, CH4, CH5 and Sky. TV shows include 'Splash' 'Celebrity Squares' 'Let's Dance' for Sports Relief. Currently touring National Theatres and Arts Centres across the UK and has performed over sixteen years at the Edinburgh Festival.

INTRODUCTION
by Producer/Director: Stephen Pettinger

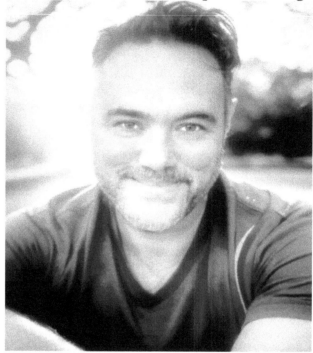

Producer/Director: Stephen Pettinger.

I am honoured to introduce Cathy Vandome's extraordinary book: a compelling autobiography that skilfully navigates the intricate maze surrounding chronic illness. It is both enlightening and humorously poignant. As a true advocate and pioneer for those grappling with chronic health conditions, Cathy's story unfolds with a unique blend of wit and pathos, perfectly tailored for those readers who want to learn more about the realities of one woman's fight to reclaim her health, and for those currently touched in whatever way by chronic ill health.

In the realm of star quality, Cathy shines with brilliance. Her zest for life has always been an inspiration. This book is a testament to her exceptional attitude to life. Within the pages of 'The Truth About ME', Cathy takes us on a captivating exploration of the challenges posed by chronic Illness and delivers profound insights with unfailing humour, leaving an indelible mark on the reader's heart.

My first encounter with Cathy dates back to our early teenage years; it was our local drama group's production of 'Joseph and the Amazing Technicolour Dreamcoat', where she dazzled in the lead role. I remember being more than a little jealous when she won the plumb part of 'Joseph'; however, as soon as she belted out 'Close every door to me' in our first full rehearsal, my green-eyed monster scarpered. I knew the Producers had made the right choice; she was breathtaking. I went on to happily play the wonderful part of the quirky 'Narrator.' It was a brilliant production and one that I'll never forget. I clearly remember our group, all under 16 years old, full of joy as we brought the house down every night!

Beyond her undeniable talent, Cathy's upbeat, energetic, and infectious personality left a long-lasting impression on me. I appreciated her talent, laughed with her in rehearsals and enjoyed every minute I spent with her.

Unfortunately, life took an unexpected turn for both of us when Cathy and I both faced severe health issues in our mid 30's. Cathy's decline was drastic; the contrast between her former exuberant self to a person who struggled to carry out everyday tasks was heartbreaking. I could empathise with her struggles, as many mirrored my own, from battling daily debilitating symptoms, a complete loss of vitality, being unable to work, facing disbelief from doctors, enduring prolonged isolation, and the breakdown of close relationships with those who couldn't comprehend our behaviour. Both our paths serve as a poignant reminder of life's unpredictability and how chronic illness can cruelly strip us of everything.

Yet, Cathy, despite her physical and mental anguish, chose not to succumb to victimhood. Instead, alongside her loving partner Mark Singleton, she dedicated herself to understanding her condition, bravely undergoing experimental treatments (before finding Dr Raymond Perrin, a specialist in the field of ME/CFS), and was always so thoughtful about others, extending a helping hand to others in need. Through her own story, she organically sheds light on the shortcomings of the Western healthcare system as it struggles to address the complexities of chronic conditions that remain largely misunderstood. As you embark on this gem, prepare to delve into a world that's thankfully unknown to many; it's painful to read at times, yet profoundly essential to understand. Cathy's words transcend the ink on the paper; they open a portal to emotions, thoughts, and experiences that will resonate with all of us touched by chronic illness.

Cathy clearly poured her heart and soul into this book, offering an extraordinary account of chronic illness that evokes tears and smiles. The narrative will resonate with all those battling chronic illness, their dedicated caregivers and the family and friends who love them, but struggle to understand. May Cathy's courageous story inspire her readers, showcasing the enduring power of courage, laughter, and the indomitable British spirit of 'just getting on with it.' Cathy's dynamic and brave spirit has always been something to behold, but when I finished the last page of this book, my respect and understanding of her journey was even more profound. Sometimes, the world views those of us who struggle with chronic ill health as weak or dramatic; it's something we all face, however, through this book, it's clear that actually, many of us are the very strongest as we keep battling forwards armed with just a smile and our grit, despite our pain.

It is with great enthusiasm that I wholeheartedly recommend The Truth About ME. It is the book I wish I had written and should have written, but typical Cathy, she's not just about talking, she's about actions and doing her part to help the world! On second thoughts...maybe my green-eyed 14-year-old monster is back after all....

Stephen Pettinger – Television and Documentary Producer/Director – USA/UK/TV

Credits include BBC 1 'Watchdog' with Anne Robinson; 'Value for Money'; 'Watchdog Healthcheck'; 'Crimewatch UK' and its spin-off, 'Crimewatch

Daily', plus a BBC Documentary filmed in Orlando, Florida. USA New York City. TV credits include the award-winning documentary, 'America Unchained', critically acclaimed, 'Tim Gunn's Guide to Style', the hit Fox show 'Nanny 911', highly rated 'Wifeswap, USA' for ABC and 'American Pickers' on history, executive producer on Jamie Oliver's 'Dream School USA', 'Dr K's Exotic Animal ER' for National Geographic, Children's TV 'Get Out of My Room' for NBC and 'Family Reboot' for Disney Plus.

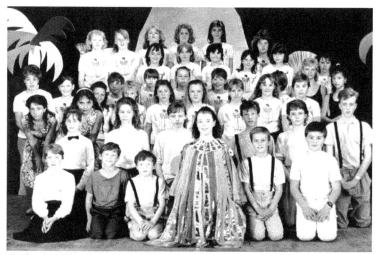

Catherine Vandome aged 14, as 'Joseph', in 'Joseph and the Amazing Technicolor Dreamcoat' with Stephen Pettinger as the 'Narrator', in the Junior Hall Players production, directed by Carol Buckley.

PREFACE
A Tribute to Jessie J by a Jessie J tribute…

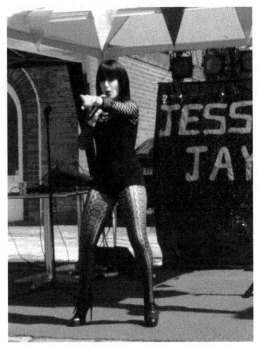

Catherine Vandome as a 'Jessie J Tribute Act' at the 'Queen's Jubilee Street Party' performing on Northway, the very street she grew up on, in her hometown of Preston, in June 2012.

Life is not about the PRICETAG, it is about the DOMINO effect of doing good for others, especially in the face of adversity. STAND UP for what you believe in and tell your truth. Never give up hope, shine a FLASHLIGHT on your future and look for the RAINBOW up ahead. MAMA KNOWS BEST in many situations, but understand that NOBODY'S PERFECT, and what is most important in life is being true to WHO YOU ARE. Fill your world with joy, and ask yourself WHO'S LAUGHING NOW, as you explode into the room with a BANG BANG, healthier and stronger than ever before, and notice the LASER LIGHT illuminating your path, as you are powerful enough to DO IT LIKE A DUDE…

"I nearly died so that I could learn to live" - Catherine Vandome

Everyone has a story to tell and none more valuable than the next. Not everyone is fortunate enough to be able to tell their story and I feel blessed that you have allowed me this opportunity to be heard. Often when we lose everything that we think matters, we are forced to become conscious and appreciate what really matters most in life.

I had my conscious awakening at age 39, when I suddenly collapsed off-stage, became bed-bound and nearly died of long-term severe ME and fibromyalgia, plus carbon monoxide poisoning, in my home in Preston, Lancashire. That is 'up north' for anyone in London using Google Earth, or just call it Manchester, for any Americans, that's close enough.

I was an independent Type 'A' personality; excitable, outgoing and a highly active entertainer working on stage throughout the world as a stand-up comedian and musical theatre entertainer. I didn't say I was funny, I said I was working!

By day, I was the managing director of my own children's theatre school called, The Sparkle Theatre School, and by night I was performing worldwide in numerous venues including theatres, comedy clubs, army barracks, hotels, variety clubs, circus tents, and cruise ships, or indeed anywhere that would have me.

I trained regularly with a personal trainer at my local gym and routinely walked my little dog Tinker, at least two and a half miles per day. In my rest time I would go to a Zumba class.

It was normal to go to bed at 2am after being on stage, after oftentimes driving a six hour round trip, to then get up at 5am to write my next show.

At the same time as running two businesses, I had just climbed over the London 02...for pleasure, auditioned for a new TV agent and had received a casting for a role in *Peaky Blinders* as a 'vomiting prostitute'...which would have been 'the pinnacle of my career!' as well as finishing painting thirty garden fences and all my indoor home furniture and in all seriousness, I can say that I was quite literally "On my last leg!"

This book explores my personal exciting life journey, working on stage as a stand-up comedian and musical theatre entertainer with undiagnosed ME, gradually progressing over time in severity and it explains scientifically why ME happens and my own personal journey to recovery.

I have written this book as a 'thank you' to Neuroscientist and registered Osteopath Dr Raymond Perrin, with a PhD in Biosciences specialising in ME/CFS and fibromyalgia, who has devoted over 35 years of his life's work to the diagnosis and treatment of this condition.

Having saved so many lives and worked alongside world leading scientists and medical professionals in the field of ME, I believe that Dr Perrin has the best scientific understanding of the condition to date.

I promised Dr Perrin that, "If he manages to save my life, I will spend the rest of my life thanking him"... so he changed his phone number!

I went in search of a diagnosis and a treatment for the most controversial illness ever recorded in history. A health condition that didn't exist, and had no cure. Everyone kept telling me to get out of my wheelchair and walk. I had no idea that so many of Jesus' disciples worked for the NHS!

I am so grateful for having had the full support throughout the years I spent in bed, campaigning through Parliament, from my Conservative MP the

Secretary of State for Defence and Head of Ministry for Defence from (2019 to 2023); The Rt Hon Sir Ben Wallace, and his exceptional Chief of Staff, Zoe Dommett. Thanks to all their help in supporting my mission to raise awareness of ME, in sharing my weekly email correspondence over the years, with PM's, Ministers, MP's, Health Secretaries, NICE, NHS England, medical professionals, scientists and specialists in the field of ME.

Thank you also for taking the time to meet Dr Perrin and myself in Parliament in October 2017, with our mission to support the ME community in encouraging an update and change to the NHS NICE guidelines for the diagnosis and treatment of ME.

Our objective was to change the condition ME from being misdiagnosed as a psychological condition to a physical condition and to look to include Dr Perrin's aid to diagnosis and treatment within the NHS NICE guidelines, in order that ME patients everywhere can get access to the right treatment and support, in order to have the best chances of recovery.

I write this book in memory of the millions of lives that have been lost to this disease, with the intent that my story will bring hope to people all over the world, that there is an actual aid to diagnosis and an available treatment offered worldwide.

This book is also a self-help guide and a support for the millions of children and adult ME patients globally, described as the 'millions missing', who are not only living with this chronic debilitating condition, but many of whom are unsupported and not believed to be genuinely sick. You are all my fellow Magnanimous Empaths!

Thank you to Dr Nigel Speight, one of the UK's leading Paediatricians in the field of ME, for your kind contribution to my book, and for everything you have done to help save ME children's lives from medical maltreatment over the years.

I dedicate this book to D.I. Groombridge from the Lancashire Constabulary, who was instrumental in supporting my recovery journey, and who sadly lost his life in 2020. DI Groombridge dedicated his life's work within the Constabulary to supporting victims of abuse and assault crimes. Thanks to his dedication into these criminal investigations, justice was achieved in a number of my personal cases.

This book is also in loving memory of Mr James Singleton (BSc, Dip Psych, C Psychol, AFBPs) Head of Clinical Psychology and Consultant Clinical Psychologist at Royal Preston Hospital (retd and now deceased), who sadly lost his life in 2021. In his lifetime's work as a psychologist helping patients, he never once doubted that ME was a physical condition and not a psychological condition, and he was honoured to meet Dr Raymond Perrin and thank him for everything he has done to help so many.

A very special thank you to my loving partner Mark Singleton, son of James Singleton, who supported me through the most difficult time in my life, in spite of his own health issues, and alongside his own recovery journey from long term ME with Dr Raymond Perrin.

Mark carried me through and literally carried me on his back when I couldn't walk, and I couldn't have made it this far without his love, kindness and support. Thanks to his own recovery with Dr Perrin, Mark is now a qualified Perrin Practitioner, who after working at The Perrin Clinic with Dr Perrin, is now at The Fulwood Therapy Centre in Fulwood, Preston, using 'The Perrin Technique' treatment to help others to recover from ME.

A huge thank you to Elaine Coleman, the Perrin Clinic manager, and all my kind-hearted friends and family and carers, who have supported me through this past decade of my recovery journey with ME.

Thank you also to all the incredible people included within my book, who took the time to write enlightening testimonials in support of the truth about ME, providing evidence of my previously excitable and highly energetic character, who did not suffer from the all too readily diagnosed ME as anxiety or depression. These eyewitness accounts are invaluable in confirming to the reader that all of the events I have been through, are historically factual, in leading up to my diagnosis of 'long-term very severe ME'.

A special thank you to Stand-up Comedian Patrick Monahan, one of the funniest and most genuine-hearted comedians on the circuit, for writing my book's Preface, and to Producer/Director Stephen Pettinger for your very kind support and words of wisdom in writing my book's Introduction.

A big thank you to my friends Mark Tedin and Roz Dunning, who were by my side over the preceding years leading to my eventual collapse in 2014. Roz was an incredible mentor and support to me, at a very challenging time, and Mark was by my side assisting me, particularly when I was about to start my 80's Diva show in a packed hotel and I couldn't remember how to plug my PA equipment into a plug socket!

As I entered the stage, I suddenly forgot every single song lyric, as well as my mini skirt. Mark encouragingly sat out front and mimed the words to me, but accidentally started with the second verse first, by which time I hadn't got a clue what was going on and thankfully the inebriated audience were more focused on my costume, or lack of, rather than my vocals.

A special thank you to my friend Sarah Flanagan, who had to choose when I collapsed whether I was acting or genuinely sick, for I was working as an actress...and then I was being diagnosed as an actress! I am so pleased that she believed me, and she has stayed loyally by my side throughout as a carer and a support and like my partner Mark Singleton and my little dog, Tinker, they have all endured a decade of ME!

Finally, a very special thank you to you the reader, for taking the time to read my book. I tell my story so that it never happens again to anyone else, and I hope it both entertains you and helps you in some way, if only to be grateful that you're you... and not me!

We all deserve the chance that I have been given to recover, because at its worst living with ME is not living... it is surviving.

I didn't need encouraging to "Start"... I needed telling to "Stop!". We ME patients must not rev our engines to speed up, we must put the brakes on to slow down. I challenge anyone after reading this book, to still think that ME patients are 'malingerers' and 'lazy' and that it is just; 'All in the mind.' I am exhausted just writing about how much I physically did!

Most importantly, we must understand that ME can happen to absolutely 'anybody'. Forgive the very people, who do not believe us today, for they may be the same people needing our support tomorrow.

However, I do believe that 'Laughter is the best medicine' alongside Dr Perrin, and without doubt humour and positivity are integral to healing. It's thanks to Dr Perrin that I am alive today…so it's all his fault!

I met my amazing friend Cathy, when my daughter joined the Sparkle Theatre School around ten years ago in 2010.

Rachel had a great time at her drama classes, they were such fun. She loved playing drama games and rehearsing for shows with her friends. She could truly 'Sparkle' and be herself.

Cathy always put her heart and soul into every session, caring more about the children in her care than she did about herself.

This all seemed to come to a head at the end of Cathy's Jessie J concert, where all the children were able to sing and dance with 'Jessie J (aka Cathy!).

I remember seeing the curtains close on stage as they did and Cathy looked round at all the children with an expression of sheer exhaustion. I later found out that she had collapsed behind the curtain and had to be carried home, unable to move. This was to be a repeating pattern for Cathy, which eventually transpired to be ME, a devastating illness that has left her virtually housebound for years, as she fights for her recovery.

Cathy is an inspiration to all those who know her. Her bravery and strength are admirable. Against all the odds, she has not let this disease defeat her and she continues to give to everyone around her, telling her story to help and encourage those who also suffer from ME.

Sarah Flanagan - Teacher and Friend

After a lifetime of working on stage, in February 2014 my fast-paced, active, busy, whirlwind life as I had known it, was about to change forever. Here is my truth and *The Truth About ME…*

CHAPTER ONE: Undiagnosed ME
There's no business like show business!

"When we are no longer able to change a situation, we are challenged to change ourselves" - Viktor E. Frankl - 'Man's Search for Meaning'.

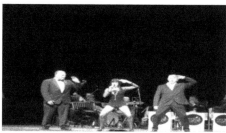

Catherine Vandome performing with 'The Ronnie Scott's Jazz Orchestra', Stand-up Comedian Phil Cool, and Peter Long the Musical Director of 'The Ronnie Scott's Jazz Orchestra', at The Charter Theatre Preston's 'Big Guild Gig' in 2012.

During 2008, a friend asked if I could spare some time to record a short CD for a friend of his, who wanted to make a present of a vocal CD for her mum and dad's special anniversary. We agreed to meet again the following week and got along just great ...a friendship was born. I had been amazed by Cathy's enthusiasm and the sheer pace at which she lived her life... a resident singer in a Blackpool hotel, proprietor and principal teacher in her own 'Sparkle' performing arts academy, and a massively positive outlook on all things theatre and performing.

In 2009, St. Catherine's Hospice key fundraiser Maureen Nickson, asked me if I could produce a 25-track double CD to celebrate St. Catherine's twenty-five years in existence, which would be celebrated in 2010. I mentioned the project to Cathy... best thing I ever did!

Cathy's work ethic and determination to help produce a winning CD was truly amazing. Not only did she contribute two solo tracks, she recruited other young people Craig Worsley, Mark Tedin, Rachel Hall and Dave Galbraith, who contributed group and solo numbers to the project.

She was happy to work tirelessly on behalf of other people. Cathy's work ethic and determination to help produce a winning charity CD for St Catherine's Hospice was truly amazing. I have never known anyone work so hard for a cause. In the event, with the help of track sponsors and CD sales, we raised £15,000 for St Catherine's from the project. Indeed, during the first week of its release in April 2010 our CD sold more copies than the HMV shop in Preston sold of the newly released album, 'Elvis' greatest hits'!

The last time I had the delight to work with Cathy was when I invited her to perform at the 'Big Guild Gig' in the Charter Theatre Preston, as part of the

City's Guild week celebrations. In true Cathy fashion, Cathy involved Phil Cool and the leader of the Ronnie Scott's Jazz Orchestra in a hilarious spoof cover of Jessie J's 'Do it like a Dude'- priceless.

For me, it is sad to see someone so absolutely full of life and happy to work tirelessly on behalf of other people so bruised and battered by ME. Knowing Cathy she WILL come through it and regain that incredible energy that makes her so special. Love you Cathy, always will.

Tony Cross - Producer

I step out into the spotlight with unflappable confidence, drinking in the surroundings of the brightly lit Proscenium Arch stage and the packed tiered audience, now in shadow. Head lifted, I walk boldly towards front-centre stage whilst singing into my microphone and position myself ahead of the Ronnie Scott's Jazz Orchestra.

Encouraging everyone to join in, I smile broadly and gesticulate with open arms on each chorus. I feel instantly connected to the diverse audience, through their warmth and generosity to participate.

I sense a two-way connection with the audience, enjoying the pleasurable feedback loop as both performer and spectator become one. I feel honoured to be a part of the experience.

As my opening number ends, I begin ad-libbing and chatting directly to the audience, whilst I introduce fellow professionals Peter Long the musical director of The Ronnie Scott's Jazz Orchestra, from stage right, and stand-up comedian Phil Cool, from stage left. Each man enters the stage with understandable trepidation, unsure as to what I have planned for them.

Uncertain of how this improvised comedy routine will unfold, I begin to direct them both to join in with some choreographed dance steps. As I introduce the number to them, I include the audience in the patter.

Like all live theatre, the outcome is uncertain and the success of the number is unknown. This is the 'pure joy' of the stage and in particular of stand-up comedy. One thing that *is* certain is that this experience produces copious amounts of adrenaline and adrenaline is addictive. My job is not only nail biting and terrifying, it is also exciting and addictive.

As the number unfolds, Peter and Phil steal the show with their hilarious improvised escapades alongside me, as crowd pleasing backing dancers. They make the number a huge success! Thunderous applause and laughter fills the auditorium, as I thank my guests for their talents, and wave goodbye to the grateful audience. As I exit stage left, I hear the compare shout into the microphone "Cathy Vandome! Follow that!"

As soon as I am in the wings, I start gasping for air through burning lungs. I feel as though I have not taken a breath for the entire duration of my performance. I am soaked to the skin with sweat and hurriedly remove the tight wig from my burning, hot head. My limbs ache and I put my lower back and neck pain down to my excessively high energy performance. I blame my sudden loss of balance, teetering backwards, alongside my dizziness, on my ridiculously high silver sequined stiletto heels. I hold onto the large black patent banister with ice cold fingers and cautiously make my way down four flights of cold, concrete stairs into the dressing room. As I make my descent, the adrenaline stops coursing through my veins. My body begins to shake and my teeth chatter uncontrollably.

I feel suddenly subdued from the adrenaline-fuelled high of the stage, which is now starkly contrasted by the pitiful low of reality. My overconfident persona ceases and my inner critical voice fires up. In spite of the audience's warm reception and resonating laughter, self-doubt takes over my mind.

I believe that I have not performed well enough and that I have failed. I feel that I have let myself down in my own hometown and made myself a laughingstock for all the wrong reasons. My emotions are erratic and after enjoying such a rush of excitement on stage, I now desperately want to cry. I put it down to the usual post-performance come down, after experiencing such a high. I am so tired. I am beyond tired. I didn't sleep last night. I have not slept properly in years.

I am absolutely exhausted and yet wound up like a tight spring. What is wrong with me? There is something seriously wrong with me. I cannot go on like this, but I must. 'The show must go on…'.

And with that, I am called back onto the stage for the full cast finale number, 'Is This the Way to Amarillo'. We close the show with the brilliant Headline Singer and Musician Tony Christie, alongside an incredible cast and a highly appreciative audience. All the productions credit goes to my dear friend Tony Cross, who organised the charitable event.

> *My strongest memory of Cathy is doing a crazy drive from the North, down to us in Reading. She got up at the crack of dawn and got to Reading by 10am.*
> *Somehow, we had to rehearse a thirty-minute corporate show of musical songs in one day. Of course, as we were young, I had totally underestimated the amount of work involved!*
> *As we entered the rehearsal room, it was dawning on me that we should be lucky to get through a few songs, let alone rehearse a whole stage show.*
> *Also, as one to undersell herself, I'm not sure Cathy was convinced that a day would be enough!*
> *Cathy met up with my wife Anna and the cast and we started on the first song. Amazingly, without any need to work out harmonies, both Cathy and Anna sang harmony lines that matched perfectly to EVERY song straight away. It was amazing! We were able to concentrate on the staging, knowing that we had the singing in the bag!*
> *Cathy came back down a week later and we had a great gig that went down really well - all in one day's rehearsal! This is my abiding memory of Cathy. It was a great gig in the end!*
> **Edmund Harcourt - Producer**

CHAPTER TWO: The reality of ME
What goes up must come down!

"You never know how strong you are until being strong is the only choice you have." - Bob Marley.

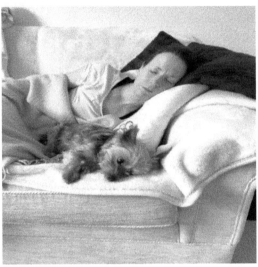

Catherine Vandome with her little dog Tinker, on the settee, living with ME.

I have known Cathy over ten years. We first met in 2008 in a professional capacity as a fellow performer in a theatre company.

Over time we became friends and worked together on various professional singing engagements, taking us around the country and performing shows.

I was also able to see first-hand, the dedication and sheer hard work Cathy gave to her second business, The Sparkle Theatre School. Cathy was a powerhouse, whose performances and children's theatre school were greatly received and much appreciated by all who have been lucky enough to meet or work with her.

I sincerely believe that I have never met a more honest, caring, dedicated and hard-working individual, as I have been lucky enough to meet in Cathy. It fills me with sadness to see the physical and medical decline of one of the best within the performing arts industry.

I noticed Cathy's problems with ill health, which included having recurring bouts of tonsillitis, yet she always powered through. Cathy's determination, strong work and moral ethics would not allow her to rest up, as we were both taught in the industry that 'the show must go on'.

Increased medical problems started to manifest over this period of time including severe vertigo. I remember Cathy in a New Years Eve performance coming off stage, being sick and going back on stage to finish the show. The effects of the vertigo were severe to say the least.

Over the following years, Cathy's medical situation gradually declined. Cathy would call me from her own show, in a state of panic and confusion, telling me that she could not remember how to set up her own Public Address system.

During times, when performing on stage together, Cathy began forgetting whole chunks of song lyrics that she had sung for years. This was totally unlike Cathy. I feel that the cognitive decline I witnessed has been a terrible tragedy for someone so highly intelligent and regarded.

When the symptoms started to get even more apparent, early in 2014, I was in a recording studio session with Cathy, laying down our vocal recordings for a Disney show in support of a local Adoption Charity Event.

In the session, Cathy collapsed as she finished recording her vocals for one song, and the session was halted there and then. I contacted the event organiser and arranged to perform the Disney show solo and informed them that Cathy had collapsed and was in no way able to leave her bed, let alone dress and perform.

Over time, I have seen this gradual decline both physically and cognitively of such an amazing performer and human being. I have witnessed my friend go from being the star of the show, to decline to the point of being unable to even lift a light A4 plastic folder, scream in pain and be unable to cope with light and sound stimuli.

I have visited Cathy in her home and witnessed her bed bound in a darkened room, in excruciating pain and physically shaking.

This illness has not just robbed Cathy of her life, it has robbed the Arts industry of an accomplished amazing performer, who gave joy and happiness to those she performed to.

Cathy is someone who simply tried and tried to power through and never stopped, even when she was getting gradually sicker.

Having known Cathy, I have witnessed the honesty and sheer generosity within her hard work, tirelessly raising money for Galloways Society for the Blind and other causes. This was not done for any personal benefit, but as a testament to the kind of decent human being Cathy is.

On a personal level, as a fellow performer, I believe that a career in the Arts industry is not just a job, it is a calling from an early age in many cases. The career becomes your identity; it is part of you.

I honestly feel that if I had suffered the depths of what I have witnessed Cathy going through, including losing the ability to perform, sing a song, or even listen to music because of the pain the stimuli of the sound creates, that I would not have been able to continue with my life.

This is why I know that Cathy is a fighter and her fight to get better and survive is sincere. I know that it is the dream of Cathy returning to the stage, in her rightful place, that keeps her going. I support her fight and hope for a healthier future.

Love Mark x

Mark Anthony Tedin – Male Vocalist and Exclusively Elton Tribute

February 2014, 7pm: (day unknown)

THUD…

Blackout…

Silence…

I awaken to the sound of an ear piercing 'Squeeeeek!'

'BANG!'

…followed by the sound of an explosion inside my head.

Arms outstretched either side of me, I find myself lying face down directly in front of my large ivory settee, on the cream woven carpeted lounge floor. I am suddenly paralysed. I cannot move. My entire body feels as heavy as lead and as I slowly rouse myself, my left cheek feels glued to the carpet.

I try to focus. My vision is severely distorted. The room is spinning fast. My sight is continuously rotating in a forward motion as though on a fairground Ferris wheel. I can see multiples of everything in view.

I can't breathe… I cannot take a breath…

My heart is racing so fast that I think I am having a heart attack. I'm absolutely convinced I am having a heart attack! Unbearable pain suddenly sears through my veins, like an electric current charged on max. Open mouthed I gasp for air, desperately trying to inhale, but with each attempt my burning lungs constrict in agonising pain.

The level of pain is so extreme that it feels as though I have been hit by a truck, broken every single bone in my body and then been set on fire. My head feels as though it has been inflated like a balloon, from the inside, putting an enormous amount of pressure into my tightly constricted skull. My entire head feels punched in every direction, as though I have been defeated in a championship fight. My hearing sensitivity is excruciatingly acute. Surrounding sounds are magnified to the point that the sound of distant outdoor birdsong has the same sound level as an aeroplane crashlanding through my lounge window. I feel as though I am inside my own inescapable living nightmare. My existence is being played out in slow motion, as in a cinematic horror movie.

Time has no meaning, and all sense of reality has gone. My brain has completely scrambled. I desperately search for simple cognitive thought processes. My thoughts are erratic and disturbed. I am absolutely terrified. Nothing makes sense. I don't know who I am, or why I am here? I believe that I am dying.

I try to lift my heavy head.

CRASH…

Sleep…

The challenge is too much. I uncontrollably crash and fall asleep. I feel as though I have been hit over the back of the head with a brick and I am out cold.

I am now drifting in and out of consciousness, blurring the lines between my waking and dream state. Disorientated, I try with all my strength to move. My body feels as though a ton of cement has been poured into every limb. I unsuccessfully attempt to move my arms to block out the exploding sounds in my ears. My right arm is so heavy that the only movement I can feel is an uncontrollable arm tremor.

The world as I knew it has disappeared. Stop the world I want to get off! My brain is fighting hard to find logical answers to my predicament. Bed. I need a bed. Where is my bed?

If the incessant spinning would stop momentarily, I could see a way out of here. Bright colours are flashing like fireworks inside my eyes and I hear more loud bangs inside my head, which involuntarily jolt my head in a succession of uncontrollable spasms. With every last bit of strength I can muster in my body, I attempt to crawl out of the living room. I slowly drag my heavy, lead-weighted body face down, across my rough-edged lounge carpet and head towards the wooden door. The pain with every small movement is excruciating.

It takes a very long time to reach the bottom of the hallway stairs, which are a short distance from my lounge. I feel like 'Alice in Wonderland' looking up to the biggest flight of stairs leading to my bedroom. This is surely an impossible mission.

CRASH...

Blackout. Both mentally and physically overwhelmed, I fall instantly asleep, unable to move any further.

"Squeeeeek!"

The high frequency ringing inside my ears awakens me once more.

I am now lying face down, shivering rigid like a block of ice, on my cold beige patterned hallway carpet, near the draft of the front door. Logic should tell me to leave the house and go and get help, or call an ambulance, but all reasonable logic has gone. I have to find my bed, where I somehow think I will be safe and I will wake up discovering that this is all just some terrible dream.

I don't know how I physically manage to climb the mountain of steep stairs, but survival is instinctive. It takes an unbelievable amount of effort, strength and determination to get to the top. I intermittently crash asleep on the stairs, as I push as hard as I possibly can, to drag my heavy bones (all of seven stone) up each and every steep, beige carpeted step. My heavily weighted head with disturbed rotating vision, acute hearing and cognition malfunction, hugely setting back my mission.

This is by far the biggest challenge of my life. Victorious and breathless, I drag my unbearably painful weighted body to the side of my bed. Face down on the fluffy white carpeted bedroom floor, I feel as though I am lying on sharp rocks. My swollen reddened skin feels intensely burning hot all over, as though I am being physically set on fire. I feel a strange painful sensation through my arms, like crawling insects are biting my veins.

I look up to the height of the side of my bed and I know that I have absolutely no possible amount of energy or strength left to get myself up there.

I have pushed my confused mind and exhausted body to the absolute max, and I have used up every last bit of strength I can find to climb the stair mountain. Without warning, I involuntarily surrender to sleep, faced down on the bedroom floor. I rouse again, and I am so mentally spaced out, that I believe that someone will find me and rescue me. I live alone, so the reality of that belief is absurd. My severe brain malfunction prevents me from thinking of moving. I completely shut down and I pass out once again on the floor. My bed is safety but I am spent. Time passes, and I wake up on the floor, still in total confusion, and I attempt to focus on the enormous bed at my side. I feel so small compared to the size of the bed. Every time I stop moving and fall asleep, I somehow recharge my energy batteries slightly, and I can move a little bit once again. I take this opportunity to achieve the final part of my mission, to get myself up and into my king-sized bed.

How I physically manage to get my lead-weighted body up and into my bed remains a mystery. Once in bed, with burning lungs, I pass out. I am physically unable to move at all now. I cannot even turn my head on the pillow, I feel so heavily weighted down.

I lay totally flat on my back, on the soft supporting mattress beneath me, which now feels unbearably sharp, as though a bed of knives is supporting my delicate bones. The lightweight cover on top of me, feels like a concrete slab is crushing my chest and lungs. My heart is racing so fast. My lungs so constricted I can barely breathe. I am inhaling fire, there is no oxygen left. I inhale short sharp breaths in the upper part of my constricted chest. This is it. I'm about to die.

My world flashes before me, as I drift in and out of consciousness. My semi-conscious existence is mixed with eerie night terrors and broken sleep, disturbed by a combination of hallucinations and complete blackness. I don't die, but I don't awaken either. I have entered an eternal darkened abyss. My thoughts and memories are erratic, disjointed and hazy. I feel no sense of time or meaning. Day is night, night is day.

I am in indescribable pain, and I am so heavily fatigued. I feel sickly drunk and cannot rouse. All my senses are disturbed. I cannot walk, speak, think, see, or hear properly. I am stuck, looped inside my own living nightmare. I believe that I have gone mad. There is no other way to describe this. I feel that I have gone completely insane! The following months, which subsequently turned into years, were a continued living nightmare. Housebound, with blackout curtains and ear defenders, I was rendered bed bound in chronic debilitating pain, following even the most minimal physical or mental activity.

Words alone cannot describe the level of inhumane torture I was enduring. I was not living; I was existing as 'the living dead'. It was so unbearable, that it would have been a relief to have died. I loved my exciting life on the stage, and I wanted my life back. I knew that if I could find the right answers to help myself, then I could also help other people as well. This became my ME mission, to campaign for the truth, and to help save lives.

The only comedy drawn from this period of time, was when I was booked in for a 'Two for the price of one' sigmoidoscopy and endoscopy, where cameras were inserted in both ends, and I only hoped they didn't use the same one. Post these medical investigations, I was laying down on a bed, high on given medications, being wheeled into an eerily dark room to recover.

"I wish I had had a baby," I slurred to the nurse.

"I have four children. I had my first baby aged 14," the nurse replied.

"Oh, lucky you. I wish I had been a slut," I dribbled, before passing out to the sound of the nurses' laughter.

Later on, I was wheeled on a trolley for an X-ray and positioned next to another female patient.

"The pain is so bad; I feel like I have been trampled by a horse," I muttered. "Why are you here?"

"I have just been trampled by a horse," was her reply.

"Then you understand."

Cathy's enthusiasm and motivation shone through her work and she encouraged every single one of the children she taught, including my daughter Sophie. Her smile was infectious.

Suddenly, it all stopped. It was as if her energy had exploded and left her totally drained. She became unrecognisable.

Sheltered, emotional, exhausted and in so much pain, I helped Cathy by walking her dog Tinker and in the second year of her illness, she wanted to get out of the house, so I offered to take her out in her wheelchair.

Well, it never dawned on me, whichever way I chose to go, Cathy lived halfway up a hill! Pushing a wheelchair up a hill with a dog that only walks when it knows it's on his way home, is damn hard work!

Tinker stopped at every gate, every lamp post and tree stump for a sniff and a pee! Giving Cathy the lead often resulted in an emergency stop, as Tinker kept pulling and yanking her arm which was too painful for her to hold the lead. It took nearly half an hour to do what would have been a ten-minute walk.

But in true Cathy sense, she would not be beaten by the condition. I would have given up a long time ago, but Cathy's value of life has made her a fighter, her motto must be, 'If at first you don't succeed, try, try again.

Julie Cartwright – Sparkle Theatre School Parent and Barber

CHAPTER THREE: Diagnosis of ME
Miracle on 83 Whittaker Lane!
(The Perrin Clinic)

"I will apply dietetic measures for the benefit of the sick according to my ability and judgement; I will keep them from harm and injustice." - Hippocratic Oath: Classical Version.

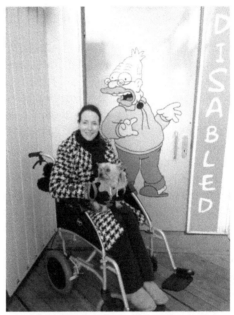

Catherine Vandome with her little dog Tinker, in a wheelchair, whilst living with ME.

I cannot and nor do I ever claim to 'cure' a physical illness. NLP is about teaching a positive mindset which can alter neurological patterns in the brain, alongside belief systems, which in turn can positively affect choices that we make in life, but I cannot cure a physical illness.[1]
Bandler – Co-Creator of NLP Neuro Linguistic Programming

[1] Used with the express permission of Dr Richard Bandler.

Dr Raymond Perrin greeted me with a warm friendly smile and led me through to his bright clinical consultation room, at The Perrin Clinic in Prestwich, near Manchester.

Aided by a carer, I pushed myself to walk with slow gait and heavy legs, towards a black upright chair with a beige cushioned back and precariously sat down opposite Dr Perrin. Dr Perrin was dressed in a crisp white tunic and sat confidently behind a large brown desk. Positioned underneath closed cream window blinds, gently blowing in the breeze from a partially opened window, he hastily shuffled and organised some paperwork ahead of me on his desk.

I slumped sideways, appreciating the cushioned chair back supporting my spine, which made sitting slightly more bearable, for every single bone in my body felt broken. My reddened skin was burning to touch, particularly my back, neck and head. I had uncontrollable right arm tremors, vertigo, and severe sound and light aversion.

My vision was severely impaired. Squinting, I strained to focus on Dr Perrin, as my eyes shook uncontrollably. Without prompting, Dr Perrin stood up and turned off the overhead yellow strip light. I was breathless, unable to catch a full breath, and my heart was racing fast, from the physical and mental effort of the passenger journey here. My head felt as though a hot pressured balloon was constantly being inflated inside my skull, and I struggled to hold my heavy head up to talk.

The relentless intense head pain heightened, and I felt incredibly sick. This in turn more severely affected my cognitive function. My short-term memory, my stress response and my emotions were erratic. I didn't want Dr Perrin to think I was in pain because I was "depressed" or say that it was "all in my mind", so I attempted to put on my entertainer's smile and tried really hard to act as though I was well.

Before our consultation, I had been asked by Dr Perrin to complete a medical and personal history form, prior to having been diagnosed by a Neurologist in hospital with ME/CFS and fibromyalgia, in September 2014 and later with bilateral vestibular hypo function (vestibular damage) in 2016.

Dr Perrin reviewed my form and listened attentively to my extensive medical history and with enormous empathy to my case. I explained that I had tried absolutely everything that I could possibly find to recover from ME, including a wide range of alternative therapies, from a range of diets to electronic massage beds, to an expensive three day 'psychological therapy course' which was loosely based on Neuro Linguistic Programming (NLP), which had professed to cure ME.

I revealed that the 'psychological therapy course' resulted in me physically collapsing afterwards, and being rushed to hospital in an ambulance with Post Exertion Malaise (PEM), and pain so extreme, that I was kept overnight and administered morphine.

I had been repeatedly told that ME was 'all in my mind' and so disheartened and desperate and blaming myself for failing the 'psychological therapy course', I had decided to go to the very top of this course and meet the

Co-Creator of Neuro Linguistic Programming (NLP); Dr Richard Bandler, to ask if he could cure me from ME.

Inside a London hotel, helped and supported by a carer, and some wonderful NLP course leaders, I was taken to meet Dr Richard Bandler in person.

I asked Dr Bandler, "Can you please hypnotise me and cure me from this terrible illness ME, and take all the pain away?"

Dr Bandler was very empathetic to my disability and condition, and replied "I cannot and nor do I ever claim to 'cure' a physical illness. NLP is about teaching a positive mindset which can alter neurological patterns in the brain, alongside belief systems, which in turn can positively affect choices that we make in life, but I cannot cure a physical illness."

I had then returned to my home in Preston, to a shocking discovery by a local plumber, who had found a broken flue pipe in my kitchen, which had been emitting carbon monoxide into my home, likely from the time it was fitted in 2006. The boiler was found to have been fitted by a non-gas-safe registered plumber, and had been slowly poisoning me for over ten years. I was told by the plumber that I was extremely lucky to be alive, as "The flue pipe was hanging off the wall and not sealed into the wall from the inside, and that the surrounding gas pipe work in the kitchen and wash house was clearly not meeting gas safe standards."

The plumber believed that this chemical poisoning, could explain many of the very severe symptoms I was presenting with, including; breathing difficulties, chest pain, vertigo, ataxia, breathlessness and tachycardia, seizures, cognitive impairment and memory loss.

The plumber Jason Griffiths, recommended that I go straight to hospital for a carbon monoxide blood/oxygen level test. I presented Dr Perrin with the plumber's gas safe report.

Gas Safe Report for:
Miss Catherine Vandome
Gas Engineer: Jason Griffiths
Date of boiler fitting at property: 17/5/2016

I went to install a boiler for Ms Catherine Vandome at the above address on (17/5/2016).
On initially inspecting the boiler I noticed that it had not been fitted correctly.
The flue pipe was hanging off the wall and not sealed into the wall from the inside and the surrounding gas pipe work in the kitchen and wash house was clearly not meeting gas safe standards. There was a hole in the wall unsealed where the flue pipe was. There were exposed gas pipes running throughout the kitchen which had not been fitted and sealed correctly as well.
I immediately stopped what I was doing and turned the heating off as I noticed that the boiler had been fitted with a broken flue pipe which was emitting carbon monoxide into the washhouse and kitchen.
Ms Vandome was upstairs as she was very sick. I called for her to come downstairs and I told her that she should go straight to hospital as she clearly

had carbon monoxide poisoning leaking into the property and this may be the reason why she was sick. In my professional training as a gas engineer, we are taught the dangers of Carbon monoxide poisoning and the damaging effects this can have on people, and why it is so important to be gas safe registered and fully comply with all the standard safety checks when fitting gas appliances.

In my ten years as a gas engineer, I have never visited a property with a broken flue pipe and I was in shock. From my point of view, Ms Vandome clearly conveyed symptoms and signs of Carbon monoxide poisoning. She looked dizzy, sleepy, drunk and couldn't walk or understand information clearly. She looked very sick indeed.

As a gas engineer I have studied the effects of carbon monoxide poisoning and they are the following, dizziness, cognitive malfunction, appearing drunk and disoriented, impaired mental state and personality changes (intoxication)

- vertigo – the feeling that you or the environment around you is spinning
- ataxia – loss of physical co-ordination caused by underlying damage to the brain and nervous system
- breathlessness and tachycardia (a heart rate of more than 100 beats per minute)
- chest pain caused by angina[2] or a heart attack[3]
- seizures – an uncontrollable burst of electrical activity in the brain that causes muscle spasms
- loss of consciousness – in cases where there are very high levels of carbon monoxide, death may occur within minutes.

I truly believe that Miss Vandome shows the signs of breathing in high levels of carbon monoxide as her symptoms are identical to the effects of carbon monoxide poisoning.

After doing the appropriate gas safety checks, I took photographs of the existing boiler which I believed had been illegally fitted, and I replaced the existing boiler with a new one in compliance with the gas safety rules and regulations.

I telephoned gas safe and reported my findings and asked for paperwork from Ms Vandome's previous boiler. The boiler was documented as being fitted in 2006, but there was no registered paperwork. We discovered that the boiler had been illegally fitted by a non-gas safe registered Plumber in 2006. This meant that Ms Vandome has been exposed to carbon monoxide poison for ten years whilst living in her property.

Yours sincerely

Jason Griffiths- JM Griffiths Plumbing and Heating.

---

[2] https://www.nhs.uk/conditions/angina/

[3] https://www.nhs.uk/conditions/heart-attack/

"I promise you I'm not anxious or depressed, I used to be a comedian on stage, my job was to make people laugh. Please believe me, I'm genuinely sick and that this is not just all in my mind!" I said defer Dr Perrin, whilst trying desperately not to slur my words and dribble, due to my severely affected speech.

Dr Perrin sat back with ease, in his large black patent faux leather office chair and shook his head in empathy. He smiled broadly and warmly replied, "I believe you. I promise you that ME is real and I personally consider it to be the cruellest illness, because it often affects patients that are highly motivated and type 'A' personalities, who push themselves to the extreme. ME is a physical illness and all of your symptoms and pain are genuine. It is still being misdiagnosed and mistreated as psychological. I have an aid to diagnosis and a treatment and I will do everything that I possibly can to help you."

I paused in shock, trying to take all this in. After all that I had endured for years, was it really possible that I might actually be able to get better?

Dr Perrin invited me to lay down on his black osteopathy couch, covered in blue rolled paper, whilst he examined me for any physical signs of ME. Seated at the head of the treatment couch, he gently held my unbearably painful head in his hands, and as I winced in pain, Dr Perrin told me that my head was so inflamed and my symptoms and inflammation markers throughout my body were so severe, that he was surprised that I was smiling.

Dr Perrin diagnosed me with long term, very severe ME and fibromyalgia and said that, in thirty years of practice, I was one of the most toxic patients he had ever diagnosed, to have survived. He told me that with three decades of treating patients, he believes "ME is inefficient drainage of the neuro-lymphatic system - the glymphatic system (the drainage of the brain) due to spine and cranium abnormalities, leading to toxic build up in the brain and body."

Dr Perrin explained that I had ME (Plus). ME plus other co-morbidities, including vestibular damage, fibromyalgia, carbon monoxide poisoning, and additional co-infections, and that would make recovery even more difficult, but not necessarily impossible. He warned that it would very likely take a number of years of 'The Perrin Technique' treatment for me to recover, and that full recovery was not guaranteed. At this, I started to cry. Dr Perrin believed me. He did not laugh at me or recommend more psychological therapy (CBT) or graded exercise therapy (GET). Dr Perrin reviewed my entire medical history, right from birth. He understood every single symptom I presented with, and not only that, for the first time in my life, he could explain the reasons why I had been so sick for so long. Everything Dr Perrin said made sense. It was like finding the biggest missing piece of a complex jigsaw puzzle.

Now in 2016, after two long lost years severely disabled and in chronic pain searching for answers, thanks to Dr Perrin, I finally had hope. I booked in to The Perrin Clinic immediately, eager to start recovery treatments with Dr Perrin.

I first became to know of Cathy whilst I was visiting The Perrin Clinic with my mum, Bev, who was having treatment for ME and fibromyalgia. At the time Dr Perrin would share with us how incredible this woman called Cathy was. Every visit there would be a new tale of just how passionate a patient advocate she was for The Perrin Technique - it was amazing to hear! It was a few months later that we bumped into Cathy at the Clinic, and began chatting. She was so vibrant and positive, a real joy to talk with. Cathy was severely ill with ME and fibromyalgia at the time and unfortunately these lively, enthusiastic moments came at a price, as Cathy would spend the majority of her days tortured by crippling symptoms.

Cathy is naturally so upbeat and for these illnesses to impact that severely was heartbreaking to see. I shared with Cathy how I had previously been bed bound with ME and had fully recovered, solely with The Perrin Technique. During my recovery with the technique, I suffered a number of relapses. As I was improving, I would enjoy the feeling of so much more energy than I had felt in ages, that I would end up pushing myself to do more activity than my body was ready for, resulting in me crashing again. It took me a number of relapses to learn from my mistakes, and really scale back no matter how well I was feeling, to allow my body the rest it required to heal while detoxing from the technique.

This was something Cathy and I chatted about a lot. Cathy is such a get-up-and-go person, that the idea of doing nothing each day was completely alien, even though that's exactly what her body needed. I found that it's all about giving yourself the permission to rest. We can be stuck on this conveyor belt of life, doing things because it is what's expected of us. But with illnesses like ME and fibromyalgia, it is so important to put yourself first.

When you are resting you are not wasting time. You are doing exactly what you need to do. You are recovering. It is always a joy to speak to Cathy. My mum, sister Chloe and I visit her and her partner Mark, to share advice, talk about experiences and just be there for each other offering support. I feel so grateful to have crossed paths with such a genuine, caring couple and despite all the ups and downs that ME and fibromyalgia bring, they continue to be a shining light of inspiration in the world.

Liv McDonald – Fully recovered patient of severe ME under Dr Raymond Perrin and Public Relations Officer for Dr Perrin.

CHAPTER FOUR: What is ME?
Knowing ME knowing you!

'Occam's Razor' – *"Entia non sunt multiplicanda praetor necessitatem"* - More things should not be used than are necessary. The explanation that requires the least speculation is usually correct. - William of Occam.

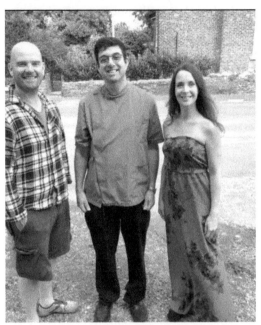

Catherine Vandome and her partner Mark Singleton, with Dr Raymond Perrin at The Perrin Clinic in Prestwich.

"ME is inefficient drainage of the neuro-lymphatic system - the glymphatic system (the drainage of the brain - my specialist area of over thirty years) due to spine and cranium abnormalities, leading to toxic build up in the brain and body." **– Dr Raymond Perrin (DO, Phd in the field of CFS/ME) - Hon Clinical Research Fellow, Faculty of Biology, Medicine and Health, The University of Manchester. Registered Neuroscientist and Osteopath and Author. Specialist in Chronic Fatigue Syndrome/Myalgic Encephalomyelitis and fibromyalgia.**

> *I heard Cathy's laugh months before I saw or treated her at The Perrin Clinic. Although I had never seen her, I knew of her, and smiled when I heard her laugh resonate in reception.*
> *When I treated her a few months later, I was amazed at how her fragile body could contain such a larger-than-life personality. I was further surprised when I*

heard her story, how could someone who's body had literally been poisoned from birth have such a passion for life. I was inspired.

Although Cathy walked into my clinic room for her treatment, her partner had to carry her out after she had a standard Perrin treatment. Treating her reminds me that the human body is resilient but also has a breaking point; however, with care, understanding and the right attitude, it can be revitalised.

Cathy's body is fragile, but her optimism, good humour and passion for living is the greatest healing she can give herself. Treating her is an inspiration.

Antoinette Atuah – Osteopath and Perrin Technique Practitioner at The Perrin Clinic

I began my weekly treatments with Dr Perrin, and as well as being my practitioner and my mentor, we became fast friends. Amidst the pain and suffering, which I endured physically, and which Dr Perrin endured emotionally, we managed to fill each treatment session with abounding laughter.

"What's the difference between a Doctor and an Osteopath?" I asked Dr Perrin.

Dr Perrin smiled down at me, as he treated me.

"An Osteopath has got your back!"

The laughter was so loud, that at times Elaine the clinic manager next door, would heartily tell ME patients outside in the waiting room, "See it works!"

Undoubtedly, alongside Dr Perrin, laughter is the best medicine. I arrived at the clinic barely able to understand my own name and as such, I quizzed Dr Perrin each week to try to learn all about his work.

I wanted to learn everything that I possibly could to try to understand my health condition, in order that I could help share the knowledge in support of other patients.

"Do you use Cranio Cervical Therapy on all your patients?" I asked Dr Perrin.

"Cranio *Sacral* Cathy, Cranio *Sacral*...Whatever you do, don't get those two words mixed up!" He laughed in shock.

Over time, I became Dr Perrin's most avid student of the neuroscience behind ME. A stand-up comedian understanding Neuroscience? Impossible! Well, there's now at least two of us, who understand it, with comedy legend Ruby Wax from America and now myself in the UK.

On 7th October 2020, PM Rishi Sunak said people in the arts "should retrain and find other jobs." Well, Mr. Sunak, you will be very pleased, because thanks to Dr Perrin, I was the first stand- up comedian to understand the workings of the 'glymphatic system' prior to its official scientific proof of existence, in 2017.

Dr Perrin explained that ME is initially precipitated by a structural abnormality of the spine and or cranium, in every single patient case on diagnosis.

This structural abnormality affects the flow of the glymphatic system (the neuro lymphatic system, or drainage of the brain), and the lymphatic system, (the drainage system of the body), which is both back and dual flowing in ME patients.

Over time the patient has an excess of chemical, physical, immunological and emotional bio-toxins which build up inside the body and certain parts of the brain, without a blood brain barrier.

Due to the constriction of lymphatic flow within the neck area, this also affects the function of the vagus nerve and the gut, for the vagus nerve begins in the head, and travels in the neck area under the ears, and leads down into the intestine.

There are two most important vessels in the body. One: the blood vessels which are responsible for transport of oxygen and glucose around the body and removing small molecules as waste matter.

The second most important system with vessels, is the lymphatic (and glymphatic) drainage system in which clear fluid travels alongside the veins. These vessels are much smaller than the veins and they are responsible for removing large molecules. Both of these vessels are compromised in ME patients. Postural orthostatic tachycardia syndrome (POTS) is a common secondary condition which can occur in ME patients and is an abnormal increase in heart rate after sitting or standing. In ME patients, the sympathetic nervous system is affected. The sympathetic nervous system controls the lymphatic system. I could feel electric shocks running throughout my body and Dr Perrin explained that these were possibly due to the sympathetic nerves irritating sensory nerves.

Dr Perrin also explained that the reason he advises ME patients not to drink alcohol, is because alcohol stimulates the NMDA and GABA receptors in the brain and these are already working incorrectly in ME patients.

Due to the structural issues affecting the flow of the lymphatic system, the ME patient's drainage is flowing backwards as well as forwards, so when this is triggered by an overload of either chemical, physical, immunological or emotional toxicity, the sympathetic nervous system can pump the drainage even faster in the wrong direction.

Dr Perrin found evidence confirming that the lymphatic system was both back and dual flowing in ME patients, by the presence of engorged lymph vessels. These are clear varicoses, like varicose veins, but clear in appearance, palpable and sometimes visible in patients. As I was very severe, I could see visible and engorged varicose lymph at the tops of my legs and under my armpits.

As the lymphatic drainage is pumping inefficiently the wrong way in ME patients, this consequently, pushes the toxins back up into the brain, leading to a build-up of large molecules; neurotoxins, as well as other large molecules, including cytokines and hormones. The presence of these molecules were scientifically proven to exist and the lymphatic drainage in the human brain, in 2017. This precisely explains the term 'Encephalomyelitis': inflammation of the brain and spinal cord, with myalgic referring to muscle pain.

We have all seen a bathroom plug, a dishwasher or a washing machine pipe when it is overloaded and it back flows toxic waste. This is precisely what is happening in ME patients. The atypical bend in the pipe (spine and cranium) is preventing the fluid drainage from flowing efficiently.

In layman's terms, and I believe that northern plumbers will understand this best "All muck is going up instead of outa' pipe!"

This back flowing system leads to a toxic build up, due to a congested lymphatic system, or a "congested pipe".

In his lifetime's work of over thirty-five years of physical hands-on diagnosis and treatment of ME and fibromyalgia patients, Dr Perrin has found that in every one of these ME patients, their neuro- lymphatic or glymphatic drainage system is faulty.

There are over 100,000 toxins in the environment. We are exposed to multiple toxins every single day of our lives.

Therefore, the bio toxin causation and overload inside the brain and body, is different for every single patient. No two ME patients are the same.

Dr Perrin said that I had most likely had this condition for a very long time, in order for it to be so severe.

I was Dr Perrin's most regular patient over a long period of time, due to being so poorly. I asked him so many questions, that *he* needed a lie down after giving me treatment.

Over the following years, I researched the scientific definition and historical understanding of ME intently. I discovered that the textbook definition of Myalgic Encephalomyelitis (ME) is described as a debilitating chronic disease, which causes dysfunction of the neurological, immune, endocrine and energy metabolism systems.

M is for Myalgia which is 'chronic pain or tenderness in one or more muscles' and Encephalomyelitis which is 'inflammation of the brain and spinal cord.'

E is for Encephalitis which is 'inflammation of the brain only', whilst Encephalomyelitis is 'inflammation of both the brain and the spinal cord'. In ME patients it is both the brain and the spinal cord which are affected.

Myalgic Encephalomyelitis (ME) is also medically referred to as Chronic Fatigue Syndrome (CFS), Chronic Fatigue Immune Dysfunction Syndrome (CFIDS), Systemic Exertion Intolerance Disease (SEID) and Post Viral Fatigue (PVF) and shares over 70% of symptomology with the rheumatic musculoskeletal pain condition fibromyalgia. Today, we also have new medical names including Long Covid/ME and Functional Neurological Disorder (FND).

Statistics calculated in 2007 showed that at this time ME affected more than 250 thousand people in the U.K. alone, and an estimated 15-30 million people worldwide. This calculation has risen significantly.

ME has historically been diagnosed under multiple different names, including Irritable Heart Disease, Effort Syndrome, Neurocirculatory Asthenia, Royal Free Disease, Mystery Disease at Lake Tahoe (a chronic mononucleosis-like syndrome), Gulf War Syndrome, Myalgic Encephalomyelitis, Chronic Epstein Barr Virus, Chronic Fatigue Syndrome and Yuppie Flu.

In the 1980's Yuppie flu was centred around the financial sector of London, with patients who were, as the acronym described, 'Young, Upwardly

Mobile Professionals.' People in high pressure jobs were reported in the media as falling ill with burnout and debilitating flu symptoms. (MEpedia)

My mother laughingly commented that "Yuppie Flu was more often diagnosed in the 'educated professional classes'", and as such it most likely "didn't spread 'up north' to Preston!"

In the 19th Century Dr George Miller Beard first termed ME as a psychopathological condition 'Neurasthenia'. The symptoms of the condition included fatigue, weakness, dizziness, fainting, depression and anxiety, and these were observed to be as a result of 'exhaustion of the central nervous system's energy reserves'. Neurasthenia was believed to be a stress condition affecting both men and women, and typically associated with upper class professionals.

Neurasthenia was also a common diagnosis during World War 1, observed by medics when soldiers returned from the war. The condition was considered to be as a direct result of 'shell shock'.

Female patients with alternative named ME, were misdiagnosed as having 'mad hysteria' and many patients had their wombs removed, believing that the cure for 'hysteria' was a hysterectomy, hence where the name originated. Many female patients at the hands of male psychologists, were told that the best cure for ME was an 'orgasm'. Typical man…they think every problem in life can be solved with an orgasm!

However, with so many varying patient histories and backgrounds, it is little wonder that the disease has baffled the medical professionals for decades, as to one exact causation of the condition, which directly links every single patient diagnosed with ME.

Until now, because my research led me to find that in the 19th Century, qualified Neurologist and practising Psychologist Sigmund Freud, observed a number of physical symptoms in Neurasthenia patients, most notably stating that he saw indications of 'intra-cranial pressure' and 'spinal irritation'.

Sigmund Freud's observations are particularly informative, as they directly connect with Neuroscientist and Osteopath Dr Raymond Perrins' scientific biomedical research, connecting issues present in every single ME patient on diagnosis, as all being initiated and precipitated by a structural issue of the cranium and spine, affecting the vagus nerve, the sympathetic nervous system and consequently the flow of the lymphatic and glymphatic systems.

Dr Perrin has found that the structural issues of the spine and cranium leading to ME, can be present from birth, affecting the drainage of the lymphatic system. First births, fast births, breach births, forceps and ventouse births, being the most vulnerable to the condition.

One of the most commonly found structural issues on diagnosis, is the presence of a flat upper thoracic spine. The upper area of the spine is flat and inverted, instead of rounded, and this directly affects the drainage of the cerebral spinal fluid along the spine. Structural issues can also occur later on in life following a fall, or a trauma to the head, neck or spine, including a car crash, heavy lifting, over exercise, or strain on the spine from leaning over a computer all day, can also precipitate the onset of ME, as the flow of the lymphatic drainage can become compromised.

Due to the structural issues affecting the glymphatic drainage, the chemical, physical, immunological and emotional biotoxins/neurotoxins, build up and cause the maelstrom of ME symptoms in the patient, depending on which parts of the brain (without a blood brain barrier) that they are present in.

The most common place of neurotoxicity is inside the hypothalamus, a small but very important organ in the brain, which is at the middle of the brain, positioned behind the cribriform plate on top of the nasal passages, and toxins build up here, partly due to a back flow of lymph drainage up through the nose. The hypothalamus balances the autonomic nervous system, which can then affect all sensation. This excessive build-up of neurotoxicity explains why all my senses were heightened.

The thalamus and the basal ganglia, lying next to the hypothalamus, are also affected badly by a back flow of toxins, acting as they do, as a junction box to communicate with the back of the brain in order to control movement. Alongside a build-up of lactic acid in the legs, and areas of noticeable varicose lymph on my body, this explained why I was struggling to walk.

Dr Perrin finished writing up my medical notes, as I was helped to walk out of the treatment room. I always laughed post treatment, as the chemicals drained out of my brain. I often looked like Steve Martin as the Dentist, in the musical The Little Shop of Horrors.

"My GP said that I will never work again as a stand-up comedian…not because I have ME, but because I'm not funny!" I laughed in a drunken slur, my legs dragging behind me, unable to co-ordinate putting one foot in front of the other.

Dr Perrin looked concerned at the severe level of detoxification reactions I was having to a small amount of the treatment. "No laughing Cathy, you must completely rest to allow all the toxins to drain out."

Dr Perrin knew his words were in vain. Asking me not to laugh was impossible. I questioned whether my excitable personality was all just a build-up of toxins and wondered if his treatments might take that away. Unfortunately for my friends and family, we found that however skilled Dr Perrin was, he couldn't remove my personality. We were all stuck with it. The hardest lesson I had to learn from Dr Perrin was to stop and rest in order to heal for, "It's not what you do, it's what happens after you do it!"

Referencing my childhood hero Eric Morecombe, I told him, "I was doing all the right things, but not necessarily in the right order," and he prayed I would recover soon, for his own sanity. Dr Perrin forwarded my patient diagnosis and clinical report to my GP:

> *Cathy originally consulted my practise on 20th May 2016 for specialist osteopathic treatment for the fatigue condition diagnosed as myalgic encephalomyelitis/chronic fatigue syndrome.*

Cathy originally presented with physical fatigue, reduction in concentration, difficulty getting to sleep, vivid dreams, disturbed sleep, short term memory problems, difficulty reading, 'muzziness' in the head/brain fog, sinusitis, head, neck, upper and lower back pain, photophobia, hyperacusis, general myalgia, mood swings, fluctuating temperature, sore throats, nausea, dry eyes, dry mouth, increased perspiration, cold extremities which are all classic symptoms of ME/CFS especially as the symptoms always worsen following exertion.

The severe pain was widespread and with added symptoms she fulfilled the ACR 2010 criteria for fibromyalgia. Her balance is affected, and legs collapse in high stimuli or high stress. She has right arms tremors and a heavy right arm post movement, so she must stay indoors and have complete rest to aid recovery.

Cathy also has significant problems with her inner ears and was diagnosed in Hospital in 2016 with moderate bilateral vestibular hypo function and this is causing severe balance problems which affect reading, writing, walking and sound aversion.

Cathy is a determined lady who has suffered from severe symptoms for many years and has had health problems probably relating to ME/CFS even before.

ME/CFS patients retain their motivation but struggle with post exertion malaise. This is precisely what Cathy is suffering from. She has the will to carry on, but her symptoms have worsened with her continued attempts to over-exert herself. Her illness is clearly severe and disabling. ME/CFS patients suffer from post exertion malaise which often means that they can exert themselves at will but suffer from the consequences.

Cathy, like most of my patients is highly motivated, but has obvious physical signs including a stiff and painful thoracic spine and the presence of tenderness in the coeliac plexus which were the most accurate physical signs in the recent NHS research project: HIVES L, BRADLEY A, RICHARDS J, ET AL. CAN PHYSICAL ASSESSMENT TECHNIQUES AND DIAGNOSIS IN PEOPLE WITH CHRONIC FATIGUE SYNDROME/MYALGIC ENCEPHALOMYELITIS? A DIAGNOSTIC ACCURACY STUDY. BMJ OPEN 2017. BMJ OPEN-2017-017521

Cathy is enduring chronic arthralgia and myalgia plus inflammation in her neck, back and peripheral joints and in particular her right hand and arm which swells up and becomes red and painful.

Cathy has problems with her ears and balance and vision, plus inflammation and pain behind her left eye and left side of her face. She is having flu-like symptoms and nausea. She suffers from IBS and irritable bladder and has severe pain in her stomach and bladder.

She has poor concentration, disturbed sleep, poor balance, short term memory problems and brain 'fog'.

She also suffers from slowness to react and slowness of thought which are probably due to the neurotoxicity within the basal ganglia. This section of the brain acts as a junction box between frontal cortical activity and the back of the brain which controls activity. The basal ganglia has been shown to be a major area of increased toxicity when the neurolymphatic (glymphatic) drainage stops.

(ILIFF J et al, 2012) which makes every activity more difficult with CFS/ME. She further suffers from severe pain in her frontal nasal, and trigeminal pathways of her cranium which are all major regions of neuro-lymphatic drainage: PERRIN R, N. LYMPHATIC DRAINAGE OF THE NEURAXIS IN CHRONIC FATIGUE SYNDROME; A HYPOTHETICAL MODEL FOR THE CRANIAL RHYTHMIC IMPULSE. JOURNAL OF THE AMERICAN OSTEOPTHIC ASSOCIATION, 107 (06), 218-224. 2007.

Cathy spends most of the day in bed or on the settee. She is unable to undertake any lifting as this puts pressure on the spine and worsens the ME/CFS symptoms. Cathy used to weight train and carry heavy PA speakers to her shows and this has exacerbated her illness.

Cathy has a wheelchair. She requires support when going into public places due to her severe sound and light sensitivity and balance problems, as well as high fatigue levels.

I have personally assisted Cathy into the clinic and back to the car for her treatment as her balance is severely affected due to her inner ear condition which on occasions is so severe that she has lost her balance when in the home and fallen. She has been taken to hospital with concussion after falling and hitting her head. I have advised Cathy not to take hot baths as the heat exacerbates her ME/CFS symptoms and she feels faint.

Cathy has problems with her eyesight and has lost her vision in her left eye on a number of occasions. She feels a burning pain in her left eye and headaches. She often has to lay down in a darkened room when this happens to go to sleep.

Cathy is still having extreme sensitivities to light and sound, hot and cold temperatures and many foods and chemicals. She is unable to take pharmaceutical medications for pain relief or eat certain foods which often leads to a severe allergic reaction. She has 'Multiple Chemical Sensitivity' (MCS). She is also showing signs of 'Electro Magnetic Sensitivity' (EMS) as her symptoms worsen using computers or mobile phones.

These allergic reactions cause her throat and mouth to swell and lead to her choking and finding breathing extremely difficult. This is worse at night when she is asleep and she also suffers from sleep apnoea which can occur in CFS/ME. Cathy has to maintain a strict diet and use chemical free products to prevent allergic reactions. This severely affects her daily living.

These signs and symptoms lead me to believe that it is possible that Cathy has an additional diagnosis of 'Mast Cell Activation Syndrome' (MCAS) of which there is currently no cure.

Due to the illness Cathy needs to avoid alcohol in any form and any quantity as even a small amount could stimulate the NMDA receptors in the thalamus which research has shown to be unregulated in ME/CFS. Also, as all vaccines contain adjuvants and preservatives, this may aggravate patients with heightened sensitivities which is common in ME/CFS. It most definitely will be a high risk for patients with MCAS and multiple chemical sensitivities like Cathy.

The hope is that with continued treatments with myself to manually remove all the chemicals and infections from the brain and spinal cord, her inflammation markers will reduce alongside her symptoms. However, she is on the very severe scale of neurotoxicity, so it may take longer than normal.

Cathy is a positive and determined lady, who desperately wants to recover and return to work. She has long-term severe symptoms and needs as much help as possible.

Dr Raymond Perrin DO, PhD – Hon Senior Lecturer, Allied Health Professionals Research Unit, University of Central Lancashire, Neuroscientist, Registered Osteopath and specialist in ME/CFS.

I first met Cathy at The Perrin Clinic in 2016. Cathy shared with me just how severely affected by ME and fibromyalgia she was. She was suffering from arm tremors, excruciating burning pain like her brain was on fire, and she had difficulty walking. Despite all that, it was clear to see just what a vibrant, enthusiastic and positive person Cathy is. Her genuine and upbeat nature is infectious and would make anyone who met her smile.

I told Cathy about my daughter Olivia who got ME aged 12 following a virus and a quad bike accident in quick succession. She became bed bound for months, unable to brush her own teeth or bathe herself. Thankfully, within a year of being diagnosed with ME, she began The Perrin Technique and it was solely down to this and Dr Perrin's advice that Olivia has since made a full recovery.

I also spoke with Cathy about how I had been diagnosed with ME too, as well as fibromyalgia, following treatment for breast cancer. I had extensive surgery, which resulted in irreparable damage to my lymphatic system. I had pain all over my body, from which I no longer suffer, thanks to The Perrin Technique, and I am able to have a good quality of life.

Following Olivia's recovery from ME, I became so passionate about the Perrin Technique that I became a Trustee of FORME (Fund for Osteopathic Research into ME) and I am now honoured to be Chairperson. FORME is a charity that was set up to raise funds for research into the use of osteopathic techniques in the prevention and treatment of ME. FORME has funded successful research trials into The Perrin Technique, and our vision as a charity is to continue to fund the research necessary to enable universal access, via the NHS, to osteopathic treatment for ME.

I am so grateful for Dr Perrin's research, and how it has helped both me and my daughters as well as many others, with whom I have become friends through ME support groups. I would implore any person who wishes to fund hope for the future to consider making a donation to FORME today.

Due to my having been through my own experiences of ME and fibromyalgia, I was able to offer some advice and support to Cathy to help her on her own recovery. As most people do, Cathy found herself pushing her body to its limit, which unfortunately resulted in her body crashing. I advised her from my own experience to pull back and to try to scale down on her activity levels. I shared with her a valuable story of Olivia, who loved to play football and who would get into a similar cycle as Cathy, by pushing herself. Olivia would repeatedly attempt to play 5 minutes of football and then crash out afterwards. Dr Perrin told her "If you keep pushing yourself like this, you will only ever be able to play those 5 minutes of football, but if you follow my advice and rest then you will be able to play an entire football match". This advice was invaluable and drove home just how vital it is to give your body the rest it needs to recover and allow the benefits of The Perrin Technique to work.

My other daughter Chloe (Olivia's fraternal twin) was diagnosed with COVID-19 in 2020. She went on to develop Long COVID a couple of months later and was confined to her bedroom due to the fatigue, joint pain and severe brain fog she was experiencing. Dr Perrin had examined Chloe 16 years prior, when Olivia was having treatment, as ME is often genetically linked in families, but there were no physical signs of ME present at that time. However, Dr Perrin explained that over the years Chloe's spine had become flattened, a typical sign of ME, due to the toll her job had taken on her spine, straining over her desk at work for many years, which affected the efficiency of her lymphatic drainage. She is currently receiving treatment with The Perrin Technique for her Long COVID symptoms and thanks to Dr Perrin she has made vast improvements and is on the road to recovery. Early intervention is key to recovery.

My daughters, Olivia and Chloe and I would visit Cathy and her partner Mark, who is also in recovery from ME under Dr Perrin. We all support each other and over the years throughout the difficulties we have all faced with this chronic illness we have become great friends. We wish Cathy and Mark all the very best for the future, in health and happiness.

Bev McDonald - Chair of The Fund for Osteopathic Research into ME (FORME). facebook.com/FORME.Charity
Donations to FORME can be made via:
OsteopathicTResearchME.enthuse.com

CHAPTER FIVE: The diagnosis and treatment of ME and Fibromyalgia
It's not Rocket science, its Neuroscience!

'I will not be ashamed to say "I know not" nor will I fail to call my colleagues when the skills of another are needed for a patient's recovery": The Hippocratic Oath: Modern Version.

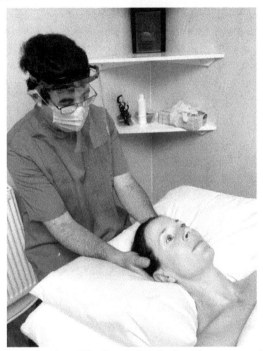

Catherine Vandome having 'The Perrin Technique' treatment for ME, with Dr Raymond Perrin, at The Perrin Clinic in Prestwich.

This chapter is dedicated to Dr Raymond Perrin, for his lifetime's dedication, scientific research, and physical support, in both diagnosing, treating and saving the lives of thousands of ME patients, both children and adults, worldwide.

> *Raymond Perrin was a lively pupil at the Manchester Jewish Grammar School where I was the Headmaster. He actually lived almost on top of the school as his parents' house was around the corner on Scholes Lane and there was a shortcut via the lane at the back of the school, which suited Raymond and his initial attitude to academic study.*
> *His real passion was the welfare of animals, and his original ambition was to study to become a VET, but places on university courses for veterinary science carried a very high tariff and were well oversubscribed.*

One of my additional roles in our small school was that of careers advisor, and he came to my office to discuss his options. In a moment of inspiration, I suggested that Osteopathy was becoming very popular and as there were not many practitioners locally, it would be a good career choice. He also had the grades that would gain him a place at the British School of Osteopathy, in London. He listened and became a star at the British School of Osteopathy (now the University of Osteopathy).

More fortunately for me when I suffered an acute flair up of lower back pain, I was able virtually to crawl into his then surgery in St John Street Manchester, and after his manipulative skills, was able to walk out almost upright. I wonder how many thousands of other patients have gained from his skills? Raymond always had a sense of adventure. His ambition to travel and assimilate new information may have been partially responsible for his drive to research and find the source and treatment for ME.

Mr Phaivish Pink – Raymond Perrins' Headmaster

I committed wholeheartedly to the weekly treatments with Dr Perrin over the following years. Although my recovery process was very slow, due to there being such a high level of toxicity in my brain and body, alongside secondary co-morbidities, I could feel gradual, incremental improvements, month on month.

"I can always be a 'sit down' comic instead of a 'stand up' comic!" I quipped. We laughed, retaining the positive spirit to which we were so accustomed.

Dr Perrin reminded me, "With ME, it is not what you do, it is what happens to you after you've done it. Just one attempt at a small performance on stage in your condition at this time, could put you back in bed for life."

"They say that stand-up comedy is the hardest job in the world... I would say recovering from a chronic illness that does not exist, and has no cure is!" I replied, as a single solitary tear rolled down my cheek, exposing my inner disappointment.

"Cathy, you are a prime example of how ME is a physical condition and not psychological, because you have the will to do, but you are too physically sick to do it. You are clearly not depressed, or anxious, indeed quite the opposite!" Dr Perrin consoled me.

"I miss my life on stage. Do you think I will ever get any of my exciting life back?" I asked quizzically.

"I believe you will get back on stage again, and I hope you do." Dr Perrin said encouragingly. "Give it more time and patience. I want you to be able to perform in shows every week, with no payback ME symptoms. Trust in the process."

As time passed, Dr Perrin shared with me his life's work and timeless passion for healing the sick. He took me on his incredible journey of discovering an aid to diagnosis, as well as a treatment for ME...

Dr Raymond Perrin was born on 24th May 1960, in Stoke Newington, London, to Hilda and Bernard Perrin. He was inspired by both his Headmaster,

Mr Phaivish Pink, and his father, who had been successfully treated by an osteopath, to qualify in 1984 as a D.O. at the British School of Osteopathy, in London.

The principle of Osteopathy is that the wellbeing of an individual depends on the external of the patient's bones, muscles, ligaments and connective tissue functioning smoothly together, whereas conventional medicine primarily treats the patient's health internally, with the use of pharmaceutical medicine and surgical procedures.

Osteopathy is an alternative medicine for patients which can detect, treat and prevent health problems by moving, stretching and massaging a person's muscles and joints. The focus is on the body's structural alignment and physicality, which are both central to good health.

In 1984, Dr Perrin became Principle of his own private Osteopathic Clinic, originally in Broughton, Salford and eventually moved to Prestwich, Manchester, opening The Perrin Clinic in 1991. He began practising Osteopathy to treat patients with a wide variety of medical conditions.

Four years later in 1988, Dr Perrin additionally became a resident Osteopath of the Holiday Inn Crowne Plaza Midland in Manchester, and worked within a City Centre Osteopathic Practice at Manchester's St John Street. Here he treated patients from all over the world, including a large number of T.V. and film celebrities, treating every patient with the utmost respect and compassion, regardless of class or status.

Dr Perrin's revolutionary discovery of a manual treatment for ME began in 1989, when he was treating a male former cyclist for the Rally Banana with osteopathic treatment for his back. The patient had not been cycling for seven years because he had ME. Whilst Dr Perrin was doing work on the patients cranial, posture and lymphatics, his physical problems and his ME symptoms improved. Within a few months he was completely symptom free from ME!

This chance discovery became the pivotal moment which transformed the entire focus of Dr Perrins future career. From this moment, Dr Perrin devoted his entire life's work to the diagnosis and treatment of ME, working alongside world leading scientists and medical professionals in the field.

Dr Perrin was used to the speed of patient recovery from osteopathic treatment, where he would alleviate symptoms and send the patient on their way. However, with the multiple complexities of ME patients' symptoms, causes, and varying medical backgrounds, this disease was to prove a much more complicated illness than standard osteopathy alone could treat. Indeed, he was soon to discover that every single ME patient was unique.

Dr Perrin was hooked, absolutely determined to find the exact link between osteopathy and ME, and to work out for himself how best to diagnose and treat it. Thanks to his patients' recovery from ME, in 1989, Dr Perrin advanced his scientific research in support of the ME community, and this became his 'life's mission'.

In 1994, Dr Perrin became a Research student for a master's degree at the Department of Orthopaedic Mechanics, at the University of Salford, and a medical advisor to a leading UK bed manufacturer, and in 1997 he became a Doctoral Student at the Department of Biological Sciences at the University of Salford, graduating in 2005. Dr Perrin questioned everything, and his inquisitive mind served him well.

In July 2005, after 11 years of post-graduate study, Dr Perrin gained a PhD in Biosciences at The University of Salford, Greater Manchester. Here, he researched extensively the scientific causation of CFS/ME. He became one of only a few people at this time to obtain a doctorate in the specialist field of CFS/ME.

In the same year, Dr Perrin became the research director of the F.O.R.M.E. Trust, to raise funds for ME. This is now run by an inspirational lady, Bev McDonald, who is the current Chair of the board of Trustees.

On 11th March 1999, Dr Perrin married his wife Julie, and is blessed to have two wonderful children with her; Max and Josh. He also has a son, Jonny, from his first marriage. Julie has supported her husband throughout his lifetime's work, for behind every great man is a great woman.

Through his extensive scientific research and hands-on manual treatment, he connected the significance of the cranial sacral rhythm to the drainage of the brain, used in osteopathy, and how this system specifically affects ME patients.

In the mid 1990's, Dr Perrin originally hypothesised, and then in 1997 explained, that if the lymphatic drainage system existed in certain animal's brains, then he believed that the human brain also had a lymphatic drainage system. Due to his background in Osteopathy, Dr Perrin could physically feel a disturbed cranial sacral rhythm pulsating in his ME patients, compared to his non-ME patients, whom he was treating.

This system is known today as the glympatic system, and it was scientifically proven to exist in the human brain in 2017, two whole decades later. Dr Perrin's primary focus is on the 'drainage of the brain' in ME patients.

Once again Dr Perrin's inquisitive mind and ability to think beyond what is put in front of him, had served him the honour of connecting Osteopathy with Neuroscience, and linking the two together to discover precisely what causes ME, and further formulating both his 'aid to diagnosis' and his treatment for ME.

It's not Rocket Science…its Neuroscience!

From 2001, Dr Perrin began running a specialist ME clinic in Bushey, Herts, London, and he continues to work there as a visiting Osteopath.

Between 1989 and 2009 a patient survey of 240 ME patients, revealed that over 90% of patients found some improvement from using The Perrin Technique, and over 15% made a full recovery following a further continuation of the treatment.

In 2006, Dr Perrin attended the Gibson Enquiry in Parliament, where he explained that Cognitive Behavioural Therapy (CBT) and Graded Exercise Therapy (GET) were unhelpful for most ME patients. Dr Perrin explained to Parliament members that ME is not psychological, but a physical condition, and needed to be treated as such. Indeed, Dr Perrin was the pioneering Neuroscientist, who explained exactly why GET is harmful, as it was due to post exertion malaise.

He said that "the ME patient suffers PEM following exercise which makes it a physical condition, and as such, any psychological therapies (including CBT) were unhelpful treatments for ME." – Dr Raymond Perrin.

In 2010, Dr Perrin's treatment was nominated by ME patients, as the third most helpful intervention following 1) Rest and 2) Pacing for ME patients, by the ME Association Charity, whose medical advisor was Dr Charles Shephard.

The Perrin Technique was the only highly ranked 'treatment' available to ME patients. Every other option on the list offered to patients, was a supporting therapy and not an actual recovery treatment. In the same year, Dr Perrin became an Ambassador to England for the International Association of CFS/ME, as well as the Vice Patron of the British School of Osteopathy (now the University College of Osteopathy) in London.

Dr Perrin holds a large number of Honorary Positions, including being Honorary Clinical Research Fellow at the School of Health Sciences, Faculty of Biology, Medicine and Health, The University of Manchester, Honorary Senior Lecture at the Allied Health Professions Research Unit, University of Central Lancashire.

He is also an appointed Member of the Scientific Committee for 2nd, 3rd, and 4th World Congress on Neurobiology and Psychopharmacology, plus the European Association of Psychiatrists' Annual Conference in Greece.

Dr Perrin has been invited to lecture internationally at the CFS/ME Conference in Florida and New York, and he is invited to guest lecture extensively to ME patient groups and charities worldwide. He has also been a Visiting Lecturer at numerous venues including at The University College of Osteopathy in London.

Dr Perrin has hosted worldwide Seminars on the Osteopathic diagnosis and treatment of CFS/ME, over many years, most notably with Professor Basant Puri in 2006 and 2007. He has also run workshops on CFS/ME all over the globe, from California/New York to South Africa/Moscow.

Since 2015, he has been an International Faculty Member for the German School of Osteopathy and in the same year he was the Winner of 'The Institute of Osteopaths Research in Practice Award'.

Dr Perrin hosts an annual conference for his ME Perrin Practitioners worldwide. These events include guest lectures from world leading scientists, doctors and specialists in the field of ME.

His guest lecturers have included Professor of Paediatrics; Peter Rowe, from John Hopkins University Baltimore and Harvard, Neuroscientist; Dr Michael Van Elzakker from Colorado and Harvard University, Paediatrician; Dr Nigel Speight (see chapter 21), Naturopathic Physician; Dr Sarah Myhill; Consultant Physician in Diabetes and Endocrinology; Dr Adrian Heald; Endocrinologist; Dr Annice Mukherjee, and Professor of Psychiatry at Imperial College; Professor Bassant Puri.

In October 2017, Dr Perrin published a peer reviewed, clinically trialled, 'aid to diagnosis' of CFS/ME which was published in the BMJ Open (British Medical Journal) Open, November 2017. The 'aid to diagnosis' showed an 86%

success rate at correctly diagnosing patients, using only the five physical signs, and without knowing the ME patient's history. This paper provides scientific evidence of five physical signs, which Dr Perrin has found on the ME patient's body and one named, Perrin Point, which can directly aid the diagnosis of the condition.

Most notably, Dr Perrin's 'aid to diagnosis' can also be used to assess pre-ME patients, to detect possible early warning signs of ME, before the full-blown symptoms occur. This is a particularly useful tool for patients with a parent, or sibling on diagnosis, as the condition can be genetic. The aim is for NHS doctors and ME specialists to adopt Dr Perrin's 'aid to diagnosis', in order to be better able to correctly diagnose ME patients in GP practices UK-wide, using the physical signs. This could save the NHS thousands of pounds a year, and speed up the waiting times for ME patients' diagnosis and treatment.

On Tuesday 14th November 2017, Dr Perrin appeared on Sky News UK with; 'Massage Technique 'speeds up' diagnosis of chronic fatigue illnesses', which highlighted that, "In tests on 94 people, 86% of patients, who had the condition were successfully diagnosed. Standard examinations carried out by an experienced doctor identified only 44% of cases."

Sky News and consequential media articles revealed that Dr Perrin's 'aid to diagnosis' should be made available to every GP in the country. Dr Perrin said that he was delighted to have seen the first signs of evidence-based recognition. He was joined by fully recovered ME patient Olivia McDonald, who confirmed that the Perrin technique had "transformed her life". (Ref. Tom Parmenter, Sky News Correspondent).

In 2018, I contacted Scottish National Party MP and representative for the ME community, Carol Monaghan, and I shared my personal story with her. I asked if she could mention Dr Perrin and his ME treatment, in the upcoming UK Parliamentary debate, in order to help other ME patients to have the chance that I had been given to recover. I received a very kind and supportive reply from Ms Monaghon. I explained to Ms Monaghon that Dr Perrin is the leading scientific specialist, who invented the' fifty per cent rule'. Following his research, Dr Perrin explained that "Patients must only do fifty per cent (half) of what they feel capable of doing in each task, in order to avoid Post Exertion Malaise (PEM)." – Dr Raymond Perrin.

At the UK commons chamber debate MP Ms Monaghon said that, "There has to be a complete rethink of the medical advice given to sufferers of ME, as even gentle exercise can set them back for weeks, and, in some cases months." (ME Association 20th February 2018).

At the Westminster Hall UK Parliamentary debate for ME/CFS, on 25th June 2018, Dr Perrin was referenced as "the specialist" by MP Carol Monaghan.

MP Carol Monaghan said, "And what of 'the specialist' (Dr Raymond Perrin) who recommends that ME patients only do 'fifty percent' of what they feel capable of doing?" (25th June 2018 Parliamentary Debate for ME/CFS).

Thanks to Dr Perrin's insight, the fifty percent rule is referenced throughout the ME community and other ME charity support groups, and is adopted today by many ME patients to aid recovery.

On 24th July 2018 Journalist Tim Gavell from *The Lancashire Evening Post*, published my media article, "Preston woman on an ME mission", which featured my personal story in campaigning through Parliament with Dr Raymond Perrin and my MP Sir Ben Wallace. (See chapter twenty-one).

In September 2018, I arranged a meeting with my consultant Head of Pain Management at the Royal Preston NHS Hospital, about the success I was having with Dr Perrin's treatment, and I asked if he could arrange to meet Dr Perrin, within his department in the NHS, with a view to clinically trailing 'The Perrin Technique' treatment within RPH. From this, Dr Perrin was subsequently invited by the Consultant Head of Pain Management to give a guest lecture on CFS/ME and fibromyalgia, to the Pain Management Department staff at Royal Preston NHS Hospital.

Although Royal Preston Hospital chose not to pursue clinical trials at this time, 'Consultant Physician in Diabetes and Endocrinology', Dr Adrian Heald, and 'Research Fellow in the Centre for Primary Care', Dr Lisa Riste, at Salford NHS Hospital, invited Dr Perrin to begin the clinical trial process there, eager to start as soon as the funding had been arranged.

In 2020, on hearing that there was a worldwide pandemic, Dr Perrin was one of the first Neuroscientists to predict a rise in patients diagnosed with post Covid, and falling with Long Covid/ME. He published a letter in the Journal of Medical Hypotheses, entitled *Into the Looking Glass*, in June 2020.

In July 2022, a pilot study among Perrin Technique practitioners in the U.K. took place, called 'Reducing Fatigue - related symptoms in Long COVID-19'. With diagnosed Long Covid presenting with so many identical symptoms to ME, the trial sought to investigate if Dr Perrin's technique for the treatment of ME, could help patients diagnosed with Long Covid. The pilot study successfully took place and was written up by Dr Perrin, together with Dr Adrian Heald, and Dr Lisa Riste.

The finding's conclusion showed that there was on average, a 50% reduction in fatigue symptoms post intervention, and that, "a specific manual lymphatic drainage intervention may help to reduce fatigue symptoms related to Long COVID. Perhaps preventing acute symptoms through early intervention." (Published by Wolters Kluwer Health Inc 2022) PubMed Disclaimer.

On 30th December 2022 Broadcaster Johnathon Ross guest appeared on ITV's 'Loose Women', discussing how his thirty-year-old daughter, Betty, has fibromyalgia. He said, "It's been a tough couple of years for her in particular, but she is getting better slowly." Johnathon Ross went on to say that his daughter had been "showing some improvement" after undergoing 'The Perrin Technique', after an initial consultation with Dr Raymond Perrin. (Ref *The Guardian* Friday 30th December 2022).

In February 2023, researchers at The University of Copenhagen discovered the existence of the SLYM. (Reference Møllgård K, Beinlich F, Kusk P et al. A mesothelium divides the subarachnoid space into functional compartments. Science January 2023).

The SLYM is the Subarachnoidal lymphatic-like membrane proposed to be the fourth layer of the meninges. It is located in the subarachnoid space, between the middle reticular meninges and the innermost tender meninges that lie close to the brain.

The SLYM is reported to be a thin monolayer of cells, and its job is to prevent larger molecules from entering the brain. Dr Perrin hypothesises that if this cell membrane is damaged, this could be the reason why a subset of ME patients do not fully recover.

In July 2023, Dr Perrin was invited to the International Association for CFS/ME Conference, as a guest speaker on the subject of ME and his specialist area of expertise, the function of the glymphatic system (the drainage of the brain). He gave a two-hour workshop on the scientific basis of his work.

Dr Perrin has dedicated thirty-five of his forty-year career (to date), to the diagnosis and treatment of ME and fibromyalgia. His lifetime's work has involved extensive scientific research, guest lectures worldwide, and he is a multiple author on the diagnosis and treatment of the condition, as well as continuing hands-on patient care, and sincere dedication to both his work and his patients. To date, **Dr Perrin's' 'aid to diagnosis' and treatment is being used by licensed Perrin Technique practitioners, to treat ME patients all over the world.**

"Chronic fatigue syndrome - I can't do anything for that!" was the exclamation.

A group of students at the British School of Osteopathy were discussing their list of patients they were to treat that day. Overhearing the students' cry, clinic tutor, Andy Cotton interjected, "It is precisely Osteopaths, who should be helping patients such as these, if we don't, then who will?"

This seemingly innocuous little incident is one of my strongest memories in all of my Osteopathic education. It seeded in me the possible scope of Osteopathic practise, and of the potential to help patients with ailments other than musculoskeletal conditions. At the time I was a 4th year undergraduate student and whilst studying for my final exams, I also undertook a postgraduate course in Classical Osteopathy in Maidstone, Kent, under the tutelage of John Wernham. John Wernham was a legendary UK Osteopath. He had a link back to the birth of Osteopathy by only two degrees of separation. Wernham's mentor was John Martin Littlejohn, the founder of the British School of Osteopathy in 1917 at Buckingham Gate in London. Littlejohn was under the tutelage of Andrew Taylor Still, the founder of Osteopathy in Kirksville, Missouri in 1892.

My brief foray into the history and founding of Osteopathy is to precisely contextualise Ray Perrin in the pantheon of world Osteopaths. Still, Littlejohn and Wernham all extolled the importance and treatment of the lymphatics. Raymond stands upon the gigantic shoulders of these three, through his research into the Osteopathic treatment of the Neuro lymphatic system. In this, he sees, as they did, the power of Osteopathic treatment to profoundly affect human physiology. Raymond Perrin's hypothesis upon the aetiology of ME/CFS, has and is becoming a mode for the treatment of this condition.'

Professor Basant Puri, head of the Lipid Neuroscience Group at Imperial College London, has described Ray's ideas not merely as a hypothesis, but as a model. This is a big deal. Scientists are very particular in the way they talk about and describe things. A 'theory' for a scientist is a very big and important thing. A theory in science, is the equivalent to, or as close as one can get to fact or truth. Scientists don't use the word, 'theory', lazily.

Big Bang theory, the theory of evolution, the kinetic theory of gasses, the theory of general relativity, these are all ideas that have been accepted as theories in the field of science, which means for you and I, as "fact or truth".

A theory starts out as a hypothesis, which is the scientific equivalent of an idea, or a hunch, or a question. A scientific model is a big step up from a hypothesis and helps to explain theory applied for a particular case. So, for Professor Puri to describe Raymond's research and protocols as a model, is confirmation of how seriously his work is taken scientifically.

Professor Puri specifically highlights Raymond's prediction in 1995, that an excess of choline would be found in ME/CFS sufferers. Totally independently of Raymonds work, Professor Puri whilst MRI scanning ME/CFS patients in 2002 found a spike/peak in choline. He then searched the internet to find why this may be, and came upon Raymond's prediction of twenty years earlier.

Will Podmore, head librarian at the British School of Osteopathy was the person, who introduced me to the name Ray Perrin in 2005. I had mentioned to Will about treating a patient with ME/CFS and he said, "You need to speak to Ray Perrin in Manchester". I duly did so, and before long I was commencing my initial training in 'The Perrin Technique'. In 2010 I joined the team at The Perrin Clinic in Manchester. Over the last ten years, I've been lucky enough to be able to consult with Ray on a weekly basis. Each time his depth of knowledge of osteopathy and neuro - immunology never fails to both impress and educate me. Whilst working with Ray, he has become more than just a clinic principal to me. He is also my educator, my mentor, and my friend. I leave you with…Leaders voted in by democracy, are not true leaders. They are merely people voted for by the mediocrity of the masses. True leaders strike out on their own, they follow their heart and instinct. Eventually, in time, the rest see the true worth of their work.

Ian Trotter - Osteopath at The Perrin Clinic.

'The Perrin Technique' book by Dr Raymond Perrin: 'How to diagnose and treat chronic fatigue syndrome/ME and fibromyalgia via the lymphatic drainage of the brain.', is published by Hammersmith Press. The book provides a detailed scientific explanation of Dr Perrin's treatment and 'aid to diagnosis' and includes self-treatments. I am included as a very severe ME and fibromyalgia 'patient case study' within his book.

To locate your nearest Perrin qualified practitioner please visit The Perrin Technique website and there are registered Perrin Practitioners available within the UK, and in many countries worldwide. Any new patients or practitioners wishing to start treatment or training with Dr Perrin can contact The Perrin Clinic on email: *info@theperrinclinic.com.*

CHAPTER SIX: The beginning of ME
Born to perform!

"It is not the beauty of a building you should look at; it's the construction of the foundation that will stand the test of time" - David Allan Coe.

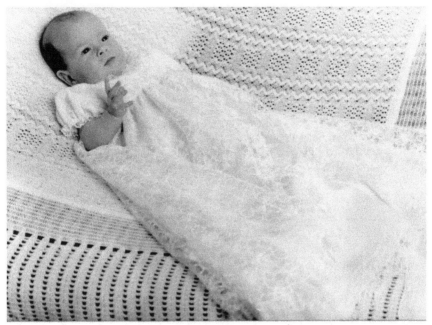

Catherine Vandome born on Saturday 3ʳᵈ August 1974, at 'Preston Royal Infirmary' in Lancashire.

"The structural issues in all ME patients, precipitate the build-up of bio-toxins and neurotoxins from exposure to chemical, physical, immunological, and emotional toxicity, resulting in an eventual diagnosis of ME."
Dr Raymond Perrin (DO, Phd in the field of CFS/ME) - Hon Clinical Research Fellow, Faculty of Biology, Medicine and Health; The University of Manchester. Registered Neuroscientist and Osteopath and Author; Specialist in Chronic Fatigue Syndrome/Myalgic Encephalomyelitis and fibromyalgia.

I invite the reader to observe through my own personal story, the structural, physical, immunological, chemical and emotional issues, preceding the onset of my 'official' ME diagnosis in 2014.

I went into labour on 2ⁿᵈ August, the day before my brothers' wedding, and I was disappointed that we would now miss the wedding. The labour pains started in earnest at 9pm and our good friend and neighbour offered the use of his car, as we didn't have one.

My husband Steve drove to the Maternity Unit at Preston Royal Infirmary and we arrived at a quarter to midnight. Since the contractions were strong, I was taken straight to the delivery room and Steve was sent home to wait. Husbands didn't stay for the birth in those days. By 12.20am on 3rd August, the contractions were so strong that I wanted to push, but because the baby was a breach birth, a doctor had to be sent for. My legs were put into stirrups, and I was told to 'hang on' until he arrived. Midwives needed to witness a given number of births before they completed their training and there was a 'witness bell' on the wall, which was used to summon them. A breach birth was an opportunity for them to increase their numbering and I heard the bell ringing, as I struggled to hold on.

Several midwives arrived and I remember thinking that if the doctor didn't arrive soon, I would deliver without him. He hurried into the room and with a huge sense of relief I gave birth to Cathy at 12.30am, and was told that she "popped out like a cork from a bottle!" I couldn't believe that we had a baby girl and I kept asking the midwife to check!

Cathy was taken away and went into an incubator in the special care baby unit, because she was an unusual birth and because of her low birth weight of 5lbs 6ozs.

Proud dad Steve arrived an hour later to see us and to hear how it all went, but I just wanted to sleep. On his way home, Steve pushed a note through the door of my parents' home informing them of the birth of their granddaughter. We didn't have a home telephone and there were no mobiles then!

What a lovely surprise it was for Cathy's Nana and Grandpa next morning when they travelled to Manchester for my brothers' wedding. My parents visited us in hospital on their return to see the baby and to tell me about the wedding.

I was allowed to breast-feed Cathy in the special care baby unit, which I did every few hours until we were both discharged five days later.

Marie Vandome – The Author Cathy's Mum

"Catherine Marie Vandome popped out like a cork from a bottle!"

At 12.30am on Saturday 3rd August 1974, I had my mother in stitches, and I hope I can do the same for the reader today. I enter the world in the most entertaining way possible, to a packed audience with everyone watching, except the BBC. The sound of applause fills the room, from the midwife slapping my back in an attempt to get me to breathe. I was a 'fast breech birth' baby, and although doctors had attempted to turn me, I was not for turning! I came out with a huge smile on my face, before the midwife realised that I was being born 'bottom first!'

After five days in hospital, with time spent in the special care baby unit, and likely on the 'naughty step' for being both an unusual and untimely birth, to the hospital's relief, I was finally taken home and then raised in a semi-detached family home in Fulwood, Preston. The hospital didn't know that in the years to follow, their establishment was to become my second home.

My father was the main financial provider and worked hard as a National Sales Manager for different businesses throughout his life, whilst my mother was a full-time housewife and my primary carer.

My mother breast fed me for the first few weeks, before I was given bottled SMA powdered milk, recommended for 'premature' or 'small for dates' babies, but I was a very sickly child from birth. My mother was a very organised and conscientious woman, so much so, that in a future comedy Christmas game, my father romantically answered a question with what attracted him most to my mother, was her 'organisational skills'.

My mother's giggling retort was that she was first attracted to his 'piercing blue eyes', and that he couldn't possibly have known how good her 'organisational skills' were on first meeting her. This brought much laughter to the Christmas table. As such, my mother kept a record of all my medical history, and my Vaccination and Immunisation schedule. This included a list of the Prophylatics given, and the dates and times that they were administered. At this time, in the early 1970's, the Prophylatics were administered in two separate doses, (twice yearly), per each first, second, third, fourth and fifth doses, as the child aged.

On 4th February 1975, I was given a First initial dose of Diphtheria, Tetanus and Polio for 'age 6 months'. Due to controversial issues at the time regarding the Measles and Whopping Cough vaccinations, children with a family history of hay fever, asthma or other allergies, were given a 'test' dose of the vaccinations.

I had a bad reaction to the test dose, and the doctor recommended postponing the vaccinations. Two months later on 8th April, I was given an initial Second dose of Diphtheria, Tetanus and Polio for 'age 8 months'.

On 10th June, two months later, I was administered my initial Third dose of Diphtheria, Tetanus and Polio for 'age 12-14 months'.

Later that year, on 7th October I was given my final First dose of Diphtheria Tetanus and Polio for 'age 6 months'. The whooping Cough vaccination was not administered to me because of my previous adverse reactions to the other three medications in February.

The following month, in November 1975, I was unwell with a bad cough, and my grandparents, Lily and Bill, on my mothers' side, were babysitting for me that night, whilst my parents went out.

My Nana, Lily Higginson, was a naturally very caring lady, who had been a wonderful mother to four of her own children. She heard me coughing upstairs in my cot and brought me downstairs to look after me and gave me some cough medicine. She held me on her knee downstairs as I slept, as she was worried about me. Suddenly, I made a little grunting noise and started choking. When my nana looked down at me, my body had gone limp, and my lips had started turning blue. I wasn't breathing.

My Nana quickly came to my aid and sat me upright on her knee, and slapped my back to try to dislodge whatever was stuck, but she started to panic as I still wasn't breathing. She jumped to her feet and held me upside down by my legs and slapped my back again and again, but without success.

Both grandparents became absolutely panic stricken as the minutes passed and time was running out, and I still wasn't breathing! They placed me onto the lounge floor, and rolled me back and forth between each other, desperately trying to get me to breathe.

My Grandpa was sent next door to call for a doctor, but they knew it would be too late by the time the doctor arrived. In a last desperate attempt to save my life, my nana raced into the kitchen with me, and put my little body in the sink and turned on the cold-water tap. The sudden jet of water hitting my face made me 'gasp', which forced open my airway. Some mucus shot out of my mouth under the stream of water, and I started breathing again, as gradually the colour began to return to my face.

My Nana had just saved my life! This created the biggest emotional bond between my nana and I, which would last for a lifetime. My nana never forgot this story, and she would tell it to me often, always re-enacting the fear she and Grandpa went through that night. She told me that I held a very special place in her heart because of it, and I remain forever grateful and indebted to her. Without my nana's intervention, I would have likely been a cot death.

When the doctor came to visit me, he diagnosed me with Laryngitis and my medical notes state that I had an "apnoeic episode". An apnoeic episode is an unexplained episode of cessation of breathing for twenty seconds or longer, which in my case was almost three minutes. The doctor informed my mother that it was possible that this was my first febrile convulsion episode, and he thought that it was due to a sickness with a very high temperature, and I was prescribed my first course of antibiotics. In December 1975, just one month later, I was diagnosed with Mumps. This infection affects the salivary glands, also called the parotid glands, which are responsible for producing saliva. These glands are located behind and below the ears. As Mumps does not respond to antibiotics, the doctor recommended that disprin and paracetamol medicines were to be administered to me, to help bring down my temperature.

On 6th January 1976, I was given my final Second dose of Diphtheria, Tetanus and Polio for 'age 8 months'. Following this, on 3rd March, I was given my final Third dose of Diphtheria, Tetanus and Polio for 'ages 12-14 months'.

Two months later, on 13th May 1976, aged 21 months, I was diagnosed with a viral infection and was fretful. My mother put me into my cot for a mid-day nap. After an hour and a half, my mother went to awaken me, but because I seemed so peacefully asleep, she decided to leave me for another half an hour.

Thirty minutes later, my mother looked over my cot to lift me out, and my eyes suddenly rolled backwards, and I started fitting. In an emergency response, my mother grabbed me out of the cot, and ran with me next door to call for an ambulance. With sirens on and lights flashing, and at times on the wrong side of the road, I was rushed into Preston Royal Infirmary.

Whilst inside the ambulance, I had a further episode of fitting and twitching, which my mother witnessed, and it was recorded as being "rather more prolonged."

I was admitted into a hospital ward, where I was given Diazepam to put me to sleep, and the consultant suggested the medicine may stop the fits. My medical record report at this time stated that I was "born by breach delivery at term", which highlighted the medical relevance of my 'atypical birth'.

The consultant explained to my parents that I'd had a febrile convulsion, and that they occur in a patient when the temperature rises too quickly, before the body has time to respond. In my medical records, the consultant described that he had "found a semi-conscious child, temperature 38⁰C., her throat was infected, but no other abnormality was found except for a 'left flaccid hemiparesis"; a weakness of one entire side of the body. The consultant warned my mother that they would not know whether or not I had suffered any permanent brain damage, until I came round. Fortunately, I recovered from this episode, and I was discharged home from hospital on 15th May 1976.

It was uncommon to have telephones installed within the home in the 1970's. It was even more uncommon for a family from 'up north' to even know how to use a telephone, but following all these emergencies due to my poor health, my parents decided to install a telephone in their home in 1976, for my safety.

Three weeks later, on Wednesday 2nd June, I was sick again with a stomach bug and diarrhoea, and I was put to bed at 6pm and as usual, fell asleep quite quickly. My father was looking after me, and due to my recent febrile convulsions, he had been advised by my mother to check on me every half an hour, in her absence. My father believed that my mother was being a little overly anxious about me, but he did as he was asked.

As soon as my father opened my bedroom door, I suddenly started fitting with another febrile convulsion. My father immediately rang for an ambulance and tried to cool me down with a cold flannel, as per my mother's instructions, and he rushed me to the hospital. I was admitted into hospital for tests and it was suggested that I may have a salmonella infection.

My medical report stated that, "On this occasion both ears seemed slightly infected. Serum calcium was normal, serum magnesium level was low, urine culture was normal. EEG was within normal limits" The consultant wrote, "I have a large number of low results recently and doubt if this is significant." I was discharged home two days later on 4th June.

The hospital consultant prescribed long term treatment with an anti-convulsant medication - Phenytoin, in view of the long fit I had encountered, and the fact that I had previously had more than one fit and a hemiparesis, in addition to being a "small for dates baby".

I started taking Phenytoin at home, when my mother observed that my behaviour suddenly started to change dramatically.

I would take the prescribed medicine at 9am after breakfast, and again at 6pm before bed. However, one hour after taking each dose, I would start screaming and crying, and it would last for about half an hour, before I eventually settled. Each day the periods of screaming increased, and by the Monday, the screaming episodes were lasting almost two hours. The doctor was called and he was at a loss as to why this was happening?

Prior to taking Phenytoin my bedtime routine was like clockwork. I would fall straight asleep and sleep through. However, now each night, one hour after taking the medicine, I was becoming disturbed in my sleep and I would wake up crying. One night, as I started crying and screaming, my mother decided to bring me downstairs, and I suddenly started having some sort of fit of violent rage. My mother described it as 'her daughter went berserk (crazy).'

I was only a very small one year-old toddler, but my family said that I suddenly had the strength of an ox. I picked up a cushion, and violently flung it from the lounge settee to the far side of the adjoining dining room, hitting the window. My father rushed across the road to get my Auntie Margaret, who was a nurse. I was screaming and flailing my arms and legs, and it took all three adults to hold me down, until the episode subsided, and I fell asleep.

The following day my mother explained to the family doctor that she believed the medicine Phenytoin was the cause of this violent fit and rage, and she said that she was stopping my medicine.

The doctor was very supportive of my mothers' decision, and said that he had spoken to the consultant in hospital, who had described my mother as 'a very over-protective mother whose child had been in hospital and had consequently been spoilt.' The doctor came to my mother's defence at this time, and told the consultant that he believed and fully supported my mother. If my mother described me as uncharacteristically 'violent', then I was violent.

My medical records on 4th June 1976 stated that I was "disturbed by the Phenytoin." The doctor explained that I needed to take some form of anti-convulsing medication.

My mother immediately stopped the Phenytoin, which was the children's version of Phenobarbitone, and the doctor changed this to Phenobarbitone, the anti-convulsing medication for adults, and I was prescribed 15mg three times per day.

I had no further convulsions at this time, and I was gradually weaned off the medication over the next two years, up until 3rd March 1978.

My mother said that she didn't cry easily, but that she had cried a lot throughout my childhood, in going through all these shocking health experiences happening to her tiny baby daughter.

I was a very adventurous little baby, and if there was ever a challenge to be met, I faced it 'head on'. One night, at age eighteen months old, my mother put me down in my cot to sleep. My cot had huge metal bars up the sides painted white, to keep me safe. At midnight, my parents were awoken suddenly, by the sound of a loud 'thud' followed by tiny footsteps running, and were shocked to see my little figure, dressed in a white nylon jumpsuit, peering around their bedroom door, grinning with excitement from ear to ear!

Not engaging with me, and still in shock, my mother picked me up and put me back into my cot. My mother was both bemused and horrified as to how on earth such a tiny little baby had climbed the equivalent of Mount Teide to escape, and she chose to hide behind the door to watch me.

Sure enough, seconds later, I pushed my tiny frame up the sides of the bars, and began climbing up the white metal frame. My mother held her breath, not wanting to make a sound and startle me in case I fell.

Like a baby Orangutan, I wrapped my delicate little legs around the vertical bars, and using my tiny little arms, I pulled my giant nappy padded bottom up and over the top of the frame, and slid down the opposite side landing with a 'thud' as I smiled and ran.

I had once again successfully cried freedom! However, this time it was into the arms of a very shocked and cross mother. In order to protect me, my mother lowered the bars of the cot that night, and in defiance, I went to sleep on the floor beside the cot. The following night, I was put into a bed for my own safety, and the Olympic games was cancelled right there and then.

I was a highly active child, and as such rather accident prone.

During the summer of 1976, at almost two-years of age, I was playing on a wooden chair swing in my back garden, when suddenly, to the horror of my mother, the rope holding the swing together snapped, and I fell backwards onto my head. 1970's Health and Safety standards of children's play equipment was not of today's regulations!

The summer of 1976 was one of the hottest summers recorded in history. Being from a family with extremely sensitive skin, my mother took meticulous care in covering me in the highest factor 'sunscreen' to prevent me from burning, a tradition I retained long into adulthood.

I was sitting upright in a bright blue pram with a hooded cover, wearing a white cotton sun dress and matching sun hat, and a copious amount of sunscreen, as my parents took a leisurely walk with their two-year-old daughter through the Pontins holiday campgrounds.

As the day passed, my left arm accidentally fell out and down the side of the pram and became exposed to the sun, and unbelievably, I was later admitted to hospital with 'third degree burns'…from Morecambe…not Majorca!

Later that year in November, I was diagnosed with Whooping cough. The medical term is pertussis; a bacterial infection of the lungs and airways, and I was prescribed my second course of antibiotics.

A year later, just before my third birthday, in July 1977, I was playing on a small wooden and metal framed slide, in the back garden, when I accidentally slipped. The rung of the step went between my legs and caused some bleeding.

My parents took me to A&E, as I was unable to pass water. I was admitted into hospital and given plenty of fluids to drink. I was kept in hospital overnight, and I was in so much pain, for I was holding my bladder, unable to pass water. At 2am I was so distressed, and I was crying in pain, because I had been forced to empty my bladder. The ward sister told my mother that it was, "most unusual to have a gynaecologist visiting the children's ward."

The following year, during March 1977, I was diagnosed with German Measles. Also known as rubella, this is an infection that causes a red rash on the body, high fever, and swollen lymph nodes. For this condition, I was given disprin and paracetamol.

During the late summer of the same year, now age three-years old, I was out playing on my street, and following the bigger children, when they all suddenly ran across the road, narrowly dodging a car which was travelling at fast speed. I was the last one to cross the road, when I heard them shout "Hurry Cathy!"

I was a compliant child and always did as I was told, and I peddled my little tricycle as fast as my little legs could carry me, to catch the other children up. I remember the car whizzing full speed towards me on my right-hand side, and I heard screams and shouts of, "No Cathy!" but it was too late. I was halfway across the road when the car screeched to a stop, narrowly missing running me over. By this time, neighbours had filled the street of Northway, and were running towards me. My mother ran over to me, picked me up and held me tight out of sheer terror at what could have been. This incident became quite a memorable spectacle on my street.

"I was just following the bigger children, they told me to cross, so I crossed," I explained to my mother.

"If they told you to jump, would you?"

I was soon to learn…yes, I would!

Over the years, our family holidays were thoroughly enjoyable, exciting, and highly entertaining, and they hold many of my happiest childhood memories. Every summertime, my parents would pack up the white Allegro car roof rack, stacked high with bulging suitcases strapped with a 'trusted' brown leather belt buckle, as my father drove us to a Pontins holiday camp.

As a child, I was very prone to motion sickness from travelling by car, and so our annual UK Pontins holiday travels usually could only take us from Preston as far as Morecambe. Twenty-five minutes was the maximum journey time we could manage, before I projectile vomited in the back of the car!

BANG..thud..thud!

"What was that?" My mother exclaimed.

BANG..thud..thud!

My father steered the car sharply towards the left-hand side of the motorway, onto the hard shoulder.

"Everybody out!" My mother shouted, hurriedly helping my two brothers and I, out of the back of the car, in a state of panic.

Lined up like sardines behind the silver barricade, we saw all of our suitcases strewn across three lanes of the motorway, and watched the scene ahead play out like a Hollywood movie.

WHOOSH!

A large truck ran directly over the top of my mother's case. I knew it was hers, as she squealed "Noooo!" recalling every precious item inside it.

I laughed. This was highly entertaining.

A police officer arrived shortly, and deserved a 'bravery medal' for taking his life into his own hands, to retrieve a northern families' trio of suitcases of little monetary value, filled with homemade clothes, teddies, and mum's precious Catherine Cookson novels. My mother stifled her scream, with her hands over her mouth, as the police officer raced across three lanes of moving traffic, successfully grabbing her suitcase in the third lane, before catching his breath at the central reservation.

"He's rescued my suitcase!" my mother cried with relief, focusing entirely on her suitcase and not the officer taking part in the horror film, 'Squid Games.'

The officer raced back across the same three lanes towards us, looking left and right, narrowly missing an oncoming truck, and proudly handed my mother her suitcase. My mother thanked him profusely, as he darted back and forth, twice more to retrieve all the remaining cases. I always wondered what on earth was so precious in that suitcase of hers? Was it really worth the police officer risking life and limb for Catherine Cookson? Apparently so!

We were the fully committed family, who likely should have been committed, that entered every single Pontins holiday competition, and gratefully came home with copious amounts of competition prizes, including winning numerous 1st place medals, and R Whites Lemonade drinks, (as a competition sponsor), for Talent, Fancy Dress, Disco Dancing, Table Tennis, Snooker, Drawing and Painting, and in my mothers' case the 'Most Glamorous Legs Competition' where she came second … out of two entrants, and was delighted not to have come third. These summer holiday camps were an amazing place for children to develop new skills, and meet new friends. I met my lifetime's pen pal; Alison Rowan at Pontins and we remain friends today.

The joy of these multi-entertainment holiday experiences inspired my future business idea to run children's, 'Sparkle Summer Theatre Schools'. Pontins Fancy Dress competitions were very strictly organised, and all the entrants had to costume their children in materials found on the summer's holiday - you could not enter with a pre-bought costume. That rule gave northern families a distinct advantage, as we were used to having to make all our own clothes!

My mother had the ingenious idea of dressing my elder brother and I, inside dad's trousers, with his brown and white stripy shirt, a large brown tie, and a circular paper plate around our necks reading; 'Two heads are better than one.' We had to parade around the circle like cattle, as the audience cheered for their favourites. I hasten to add that my father was not wearing his clothes at the same time!

This unique costume idea of my mothers' won first prize, and we appeared in the local newspaper. Years later, my mother creatively entered the same costume, and this time I was joined with my younger brother, wearing my father's clothes whilst trying to walk in lockstep, and we too won first prize, and once again, in spite of the physical discomfort, we proudly appeared in the local newspaper.

We were all excited as first prize competition winners, to be awarded another holiday the same year to 'Brean sands' to join other competition winners, and compete for the UK's ultimate first prize, though our parents were less so.

After one year's freezing cold and thoroughly miserable and wet experience, in December, within a location more akin to, "I'm a celebrity get me out of here!" my parents subsequently attempted to find as many excuses as possible, for us never to go again.

Over the following years, my parents resorted to clapping loudly for the other child competitors to, "See how they like winning!"

I can remember when Cathy was about three years old and we were on holiday at Pontins, and in passing the children's play area her mum would ask if she and her older brother would like to play there for a little while, but before we had chance to explain the arrangements, Cathy was off on the swings and the slides, and it was left to her brother to listen to the arrangements to meet again. Fortunately, there was a Bluecoat supervising the children, so at least she was safe.

"The same situation would apply in the ballroom when the children were invited to come to the front and sit on the floor to watch the Cabaret. Cathy would just dash off without considering where we would be sat or what time to be back. It was left to her brother again to sort out the arrangements, and typical of her self-confidence, she would say to her older brother "Don't worry, I'll look after you!"

"Her energy and confidence to take part in whatever was happening, without worry or fear as to what she was getting into, was very much part of Cathy from an early age.

"This confidence continued into her adult life and played an important part in her stage career. Whether it was a part in a musical, singing, dancing, acting or a Cabaret spot in a club, she maintained that confidence and could always hold an audience.

"Perhaps the most memorable occasion was the 2012 Preston Guild Variety Show at the Charter Theatre, when Cathy manipulated the leader of the 'Ronnie Scott Jazz Orchestra' and the show compere, comedian Phil Cool, to take part in an ad lib comedy sketch, which she led whilst she sang, 'Do It Like A Dude' as Jessie J – a sketch that Morecambe and Wise would have been proud to perform. It went down a treat and amidst the laughter at the end came the shout - "Follow that!". xx

Steve Vandome – The Author Cathy's Dad

CHAPTER SEVEN: Growing up as ME
School daze!

"I will neither give a deadly drug to anybody who asked for it, nor will I make a suggestion to this effect."- Hippocratic Oath - Classical Version.

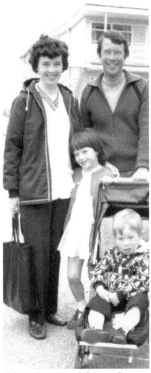

Mum Marie, Dad Steve, and brother David Vandome. Catherine Vandome age six, on holiday with her family, at the Pontin's Holiday Camp, Morecombe, in 1981.

"A skilled craftsman will have a toolbox full of many tools. He may need a hammer, a screwdriver, a saw, a level or a drill. If he only has a spanner and a chisel, he will be quite limited in what he can do. Unfortunately, modern western medicine mainly uses a scalpel or a prescription pad. These are useful and modern medicine can be amazing, but there are many more ways of helping people than just with these two tools."
Michael Gregson – Osteopath at The Fulwood Therapy Centre

School bag - ☑
Dinner money - ☑
Adult dose of phenobarbitals - ☑ and off I went to school.

I was raised a Catholic, and started at Our Lady's Catholic Primary School in September 1978. Most children in my year group were almost five years old, but as an August born baby, I had only just turned four.

After a tearful separation from my mother at the school gates, with me crying, not my mother, I approached school life with confidence. I was physically very active as well as creative, and my school reports highlighted that I always tried my best in whatever I did, and in whatever task was asked of me.

As was the 1980's schooling, I was afraid of any and all authority figures.

One day in class, aged four years old, the teacher set the task of putting triangles, squares and circles onto separate lines. I didn't understand this simple task, and so I asked a friend to help me, who for a joke told me to put all the shapes onto one line. I proudly handed in my work, and I was immediately shouted at by the teacher, in front of the whole class, smacked and sent to stand by the dolls' house, facing away from everyone. I remember feeling humiliated, because I genuinely didn't understand the set work. I wasn't being naughty.

My only consolation was being joined by a fellow August born, four-year-old school friend, Rachel Kellett, who had just received the same corporal punishment, and we stood side by side by the doll's house with watery eyes...wishing we were five!

This incident set the precedence for my conditioned fear of authority figures, which continued throughout most of my adult life. However, I came into my own, when at aged four, I was cast in my first comedy role in my first ever theatrical stage production. Donned in a pointed goblin hat, bright blue leotard and matching tights, which exaggerated my rotund belly, I was cast as a little milk maid. Holding my large silver bucket, I ran onto the stage smiling from ear to ear.

I remember getting such resounding laughter from the audience as I appeared on stage, with the singers around me reciting, "Run little goblin, run along to market and buy me a cow."

I thought, "I like this feeling, I like making people laugh!"

The stage felt like home, and from this moment on, the theatre became my whole world.

I lived in a hyper-stimulated and excitable state, yet I was always feeling 'tired but wired'. I was also in a hyper vigilant state of 'fight or flight', as though anticipating that something terrible was about to happen. My memory and thought processing were severely affected, and I struggled to retain information.

In my school exams, the teachers would console my parents, by explaining that "Cathy is a bright child, she just gets very nervous in exams, and her results don't reflect her ability in class."

Many evenings my mother would take a nightly stroll to my young childhood best friend, Jennifer Woodburn's house, to ask her what the school homework was, and to find out whether there was any information notices from school, as my mother would repeatedly say, "Cathy is always half asleep and forgetful."

On 4th May 1979, I was given my initial Forth dose of Diphtheria, Tetanus and Polio for 'age 5 years or school entry.'

Later this same year, I was signed off at the hospital and my barbiturates medication, Phenobarbitone was stopped. My mother was assured by the doctor that there was no risk of my having anymore febrile convulsions because, "Children grew out of them when they reach the age of five".

On 4th September, I was given my final Forth dose of Diphtheria, Tetanus and Polio for 'age 5 years or school entry.'

The following February, in 1981, now aged six years, my mother kept me off school, as I had a very high temperature, with flu-like symptoms.

I spent the morning laying on the settee, one minute wrapped in a blanket shivering, and the next sweating, holding my new best friend; a small brown plastic sick bucket with a white handle. I eventually fell asleep having taken disprin and paracetamol to bring my temperature down, but when my mother went to waken me, I suddenly started fitting. My mother grabbed hold of me and carried me from the settee, and placed me onto the kitchen floor, dousing me with wet towels in an attempt to lower my temperature. She raced to call for a neighbour to come and help me, who rang for an ambulance.

My medical records confirm that I was "admitted on 12th February in 'status epilepticus'. Status epilepticus is a life-threatening neurological condition and carries a high mortality and morbidity. It is defined by the National Institute for Health and Care Excellence as a convulsive seizure that continues for longer than five minutes. (BMJ Best Practice).

I was kept in hospital for four days and monitored, and returned home with a new medicine to control the febrile convulsions, called Epilim. After recovering from this febrile convulsion, I was now taking Epilim as prescribed. However, I was now becoming increasingly drowsy, quiet and lethargic, the opposite of my natural character.

After ten days of taking Epilim, my mother described me as having "lost my sparkle". She explained to the doctor that her daughter "would sit looking at a book for long periods of time, without turning any of the pages, and was like a walking zombie". My mother said that "she now couldn't trust me to be alert enough to cross the road safely."

She questioned whether this was the new medicine causing the severe reaction, or whether the latest convulsion had affected my brain, pointing out to medical professionals that her daughter had always been so confident and full of life, and that she didn't like this change in my personality.

My mother researched Epilim medicine, and told the Paediatrician her concerns, but the Paediatrician was 'adamant' that the medicine wasn't the cause.

The Paediatrician told my mother "I cannot stand over you and make you give her this medicine, but if she has another convulsion, she will have to take it whether you like it or not!"

"She won't have another convulsion. I will monitor her and make sure of that!" My mother replied and immediately stopped the Epilim medication, and as a result of this, my personality soon returned to my old lively self.

Many years later, it was discovered that Epilim had been banned from use in the U.K. as it had caused severe learning difficulties in children.

I had an electroencephalogram (E.E.G.) brain scan, which showed 'moderate posterior dysrhythmia'. The doctors' medical records state that "if she has any further convulsions, I think Carbamzapine would be the drug to try at that point. I have discussed at length with mother (who is fairly strongly opposed to any treatment) that the prolonged nature of her initial convulsion, plus the Todd's paresis afterwards, plus the fact that she has now had a convulsion at the age of six and a half years, are all factors that would make one slightly suspicious that this could occur again."

In April 1981, three months after my febrile convulsion, I was very sick again with a temperature of 104°F and I was diagnosed with Measles.

That night, as my temperature began to rise, my mother sponged my body down to keep it cool, and administered soluble disprin every four hours, as instructed, throughout the night. She monitored me carefully, as she was afraid of my having another febrile convulsion and being forced by the Paediatrician to administer medication if I did. When I returned to school, I had to be monitored whenever I became sick, just in case I had another febrile convulsion.

In the 1980's, many primary schools had sick beds set up inside the classroom, and if children felt unwell, they would be told to lay down in the sick bed. The sick bed was comprised of a dark green combat material camp bed with a wooly brown head pillow. My brothers action man toy had an identical bed in miniature, and yes, I was so tiny, no doubt I could have fitted inside that!

The school sick bed access became a little bit of a game for some children wanting to get out of lessons and have some 'attention' from others. I remember two school friends each putting their hands up and telling the teacher that they felt sick, and being told to lay down in the two adjoining sick beds. However, being sick most of the time, whenever I put my hand up and told the teacher I was sick, I was always told to "put my head in my hands and sit up at the table". Well, that wasn't much fun, and I felt left out and wondered why I was never allowed to lay down in the sickbed.

My mother explained to me that I was not allowed to lay down or fall asleep in school when I was sick, just in case I had another febrile convulsion or fainted. My mother's intentions were honourable. She was not going to have her daughter prescribed more anticonvulsant medications, just for ten minutes of extra classroom attention!

In spite of my outward confidence, I was a very sensitive little girl and frightened of so many things. I was regularly having acutely terrifying nightmares, waking up crying in sheer fear, with hot sweats and recurrent night terrors. In the middle of the night, my mother would hear me scream and come to my aid, slowly peering around my creaking bedroom door, but on seeing her genetic, deathly white complexion, I would cry out "Ahh! You look like a ghost!"

With that, she would disappear, leaving me to question whether she really was an apparition! The night terrors continued through into adulthood, but once I moved house, I never saw that particular ghost again.

My nana thoroughly enjoyed entertaining me, and would often read children's stories to me. One afternoon, she read the children's story of 'Goosey

Goosey Gander.' and as soon as she said the words, "He took him by the left leg and threw him down the stairs" and showed me the adjoining picture of an old man throwing a huge white goose downstairs, I burst into tears in fear. I was easily startled. We couldn't even open the book about 'Rumplestiltskin!' How did these children's stories ever get to print!

Throughout my primary school years, I oftentimes had to miss school classes, and events and instead have private reading lessons in another classroom, because I was unusually frightened of particular books, television programmes or subject material, and this was badly affecting my sleep. Unbeknownst to me, my mother arranged these private reading lessons with the teachers, as it was disturbing for her to watch her child crying in this incredibly frightened state each night.

In 1982, when I was aged seven, there was a touring theatre production company visiting my primary school. My teacher asked my mother if she was having financial difficulties and couldn't afford to pay the £1 fee for me to watch the theatre production in school? The teacher explained that I was "the only child in the entire school that hadn't yet paid the fee."

My mother said that she knew nothing about this theatre production, and asked what the production was?

'Rumplestiltskin.' the teacher replied.

My mother laughed heartily, and said "That was why Cathy hadn't paid the fee, because she was absolutely terrified of this story, and that she wouldn't be watching it."

One afternoon, after school, I was at my friend, Jennifer's house, seated on the lounge settee in between her and her nana.

"Have you seen Worzel Gummidge before Cathy?" asked Edith Scott, Jennifers nana.

"No," I smiled, expecting it to be a comedy.

The T.V. show's music and titles began, and suddenly the most terrifying scarecrow filled up the entire screen, and winked at me.

"Ahhhhh!" I screamed in sheer fear, subconsciously throwing my long, blue, plastic cup filled to the brim with orange squash, all over Jennifers nana.

I ran straight out of the room shaking uncontrollably, into the arms of Auntie Carole, (Jennifer's mother), who held me tight and consoled me. She had never seen me react like this before. It took me a while to calm down and feel safe enough to go back home, all of five doors away along the same street. Carole saw for herself just how terrified I could become.

No-one thought to ask poor Edith just how she was feeling, sat frozen in shock, drenched in sticky orange squash slowly dripping down her face and onto her blouse. Edith was the sister of football legend, 'Preston North Ends' Sir Tom Finney, and this wouldn't be the only time that I would spill an entire drink over a footballer's sibling, or indeed the star player themselves!

Throughout my childhood years, I was becoming increasingly sick, and being diagnosed by doctors with multiple infections and viruses, but no matter how poorly I was, I would always get back up and push myself harder to achieve my goals. On top of this, I was also having recurrent fainting episodes, vomiting, nose bleeds and constantly sneezing, with flu-like symptoms.

When I started having recurrent nosebleeds at school, this was put down to my being 'physically very active and always running around everywhere'.

A slight bang on the nose, and it wouldn't stop bleeding. Though oftentimes it started for no reason at all just 'drip, drip, drip', onto my schoolwork, before I was escorted out of the room, so I didn't frighten the other children!

I regularly sat outside of the classroom alone, tipping my head back with a bright, blue, paper towel over my nose to stop the bleeding; swallowing what seemed like pints of metallic tasting blood. (We now know that tipping the head backwards is the opposite way to stop a nosebleed!) Numerous times my nose wouldn't stop bleeding for so long, that I would become faint and sent home.

My fainting episodes were frequent, and worsened when I got very over excited about things. Every Christmas morning in church, my father would routinely seat me near the exit of the pew bench and watch his young daughter turn from pasty white to bright yellow.

As a devout Catholic, my dad would be ready to scoop me up in his arms and charge out of the back of church with me over his shoulder, before I projectile vomited in a place of worship!

Numerous times his mission to exit the back of church failed, and he would say an extra three 'Hail Mary's for our sins.

My sleep was becoming affected, and I would struggle to get up in the mornings for school. I was sometimes sleeping for twelve hours per night, and yet still feeling tired and unrefreshed.

I was upset one morning and I didn't want to get up for school, for I was so tired and always felt bitterly freezing cold in the mornings.

I told my father, "When I am a grown up I am not going to go to work in the mornings, I am going to find a job that starts work later on."

My father, having worked exceptionally hard with early mornings his whole life as a National Sales Manager, laughed and replied, "There are no jobs that start late in the day!"

With a future career on stage, I was later to prove him wrong!

In school, my passions were performing on the stage, writing, and sports activities, and I really struggled with Maths and number work.

I discovered that a lot of stand-up comedian's struggle with Mathematics, suffering from dyscalculia, which is an inability to add up numbers properly. Well, Ken Dodd and Jimmy Carr certainly did!

My A4 sized Beta Mathematics book became my worst enemy, as I was instructed to have extra tuition at home to catch up. I continued to work hard at everything I did. I was incredibly physically active, and absolutely fearless when it came to participating in school sports activities. I enjoyed all sports, and with a competitive spirit, I would always find that extra boost of energy and adrenaline needed to try to win. I did not let my very short stature hold me back.

In school gymnastics one afternoon, I jumped off the small blue trampoline and summersaulted over the large brown wooden box, landing badly with a crunch on my left ankle. This was significant, because it was when I first realised that my joints were hyper mobile. My ankle had rolled extremely far over the wrong way and immediately swelled up like a black and blue balloon.

The pain was severe and the schoolteacher insisted that it must be broken, so I went straight to Accident and Emergency, where hospital staff were equally surprised that it was badly sprained, but hadn't actually broken.

On 30th January 1984, I was diagnosed with Chicken Pox. I remember this being an unbearable sickness, covered in spots, with incessant scratching and the constant reapplication of calamine lotion which smelt terrible, and burned instead of soothed my skin.

The following year, on 13th May 1985, I had a high temperature, with an itchy rash, and aching swollen joints. For this I was prescribed Penicillin. The symptoms lasted a week, and I was consequently diagnosed with Parvovirus.

I had never heard of Parvovirus before, and I knew nobody else with it. I soon learned that Parvovirus was a disease that dogs get…which explained a lot!

In the summer term of the same year, now in Junior 4 (Year 6) I won the long jump. Long jump rules being to 'Run, jump, and leap into the sandpit, taking off within the wooden board perimeters and landing on two feet'.

This momentous victory surprised all the teachers and students, and me, because I was one of the shortest in the class. I watched the teachers shake their heads in complete surprise, making it very obvious that my hobbit stature and jumping abilities were an unusual combination.

I was also put up to try out for the high jump team, as I was such a springy little ball of energy. One teacher during the competition raised the high jump bar and said, "Right, everyone else in line try this, but not you Cathy."

"Please let me try!" I begged, and I ran up at top speed and made it cleanly over the bar.

The teacher held her hands to her head and laughed out loud in sheer astonishment…and no doubt went straight to the bar herself!

Amongst other sports events, I made both the high jump and long jump team, and I thought how much further athletics training I could have had, had my mother not moved me from my cot into a bed. The great thing about the 1980's teachers, were that 'they said it as it really was'…and they all helped encourage me to have a long-lasting height complex. As a hobgoblin, it was no surprise that I would become a member of the local community of Brownies.

My Brownie Guide Leader 'Brown Owl', was a lovely local lady, Marion Fogerty, and she was perfectly assisted by her 'Tawny Owl', Carole Woodburn, or 'Auntie Carole' to me, as she was my friend, Jennifer's mother.

In Scottish folklore, 'Brownies' are said to come out at night when the owners of the house are asleep and perform various chores. This explained why all the Brownies achievement badges, were centred around performing chores for others. I once stood atop a wooden stool, and with my sensitive little hands, completed the biggest pile of washing up I had ever seen in my life, for a local elderly lady. That night I successfully achieved my 'Brownie child labour' badge.

My Uncles Bill, John, and Paul (my mother's brothers) would keep us all entertained as children, with numerous games, sporting activities, and assault courses in the garden. As a high achieving and competitive family, we learned to try the very best we could in all things, and this passion for all games, inspired by my nana, united the whole family and brought copious amounts of fun and laughter. I was happy to make people laugh with my surprising athletic feats, and that was most important to me, it didn't matter how ridiculous I looked to them. My friend Jennifer and I would win a number of Sports' Day bean bag and relay races. Jennifer went on to become a solicitor, and from a young age she was clever enough to make me the wheelbarrow for any and all races.

As a human wheelbarrow, Jennifer would push me as fast as my little springy arms would take us, and when we were first to the finish line, she was somehow rewarded with fifty percent of the credit! I wonder how many childhood Sports' Day trophies I would have had to return, had I been 'drugs tested' for performance enhancing Barbiturates!

I was an excitable little nipper, zipping around like a mini–George Best on the school playing fields. Rounders was a personal sporting favourite, as I had great hand eye coordination, so I could hit the ball hard, and run like the wind, always aiming for at least two rounders! I was like a pint-sized version of the T.V. cartoon character, 'Road runner'.

Being a fast runner was also useful in the school playground, with popular 1980's games like 'British bulldog', where two teams of children, (consisting of boys and girls), would charge en mass across the playground knocking each other over to get to the other side. This game was later banned in schools for the injury levels, because over time teachers started to care about the children's welfare.

I was very competitive and being able to run fast was particularly useful in 'Kiss catch', as I could outrun the boys on the playing fields trying to kiss me. Some boys would wait until the game was over, grab me and lamp a big, wet, sloppy kiss on my cheek, as I protested that the game had finished ten minutes ago, whilst I rubbed their excess dribble off my face with the sleeve of my royal blue school cardigan. I can't think why these children's games are banned today, the 1980's was character building!

Keep Twinkling! What can you say when you meet a very passionate, talented woman with so much indefatigable energy and zest for life?

Over 16 years ago, I had the good fortune to meet Cathy Vandome. Her enthusiastic and caring nature was infectious, and I, like many countless others was hooked! The Sparkle Theatre School, Cathy's brainchild of combining music, dance, song and drama was born and it was so popular that I don't think she could keep up with the number of children and youngsters, that she had to set up many groups, some with two or three sessions per afternoon and evening and five times a week.

It must have been exhausting, but Cathy's energy, resolve and will to share her undoubted and natural talent could not be moved. Cathy had dedicated most of her life to that point, in giving herself through her work as a professional singer, artist, entertainer and performer, sharing her many gifts with countless hopeful youngsters, who were drawn literally to the sparkle, her personality shining like the stars we all hope to reach for, but very few do.

Cathy was never driven by financial success, she simply loved her work - it was more like a vocation to support the youngsters in her care.

Cathy's nana suffered poor sight, which deteriorated as she grew older. It must have been hard for her to see her nana struggling. Galloways, which was "her Nana's Charity', is a wonderful local Charity and I had the privilege to try and support Cathy's nana to try to help her 'retain' some of her vision and a level of independence.

It was just my job, but after meeting Cathy sometime later, I realised that even the smallest help can make a huge difference and I'd not realised how grateful she truly was. I couldn't keep up with Cathy, as she set up Easter and Summer schools for the children, freely giving of herself for so many children, including my daughter, who developed so much confidence, which I'm sure Cathy had instilled.

I remember providing visual awareness training sessions for the children aged between four and twenty, an adapting task, yet it was another privilege, as Cathy had prepared the youngsters to help them understand what it's like to live in a world of sight loss or blindness. Filming and creating a movie around the issues affecting people with sight loss was very special too, as was the 'red carpet' treatment in the cinema.

The youngsters were introduced to the studios of Galloways Talking Newspaper to highlight how people receive their news and information in different ways, including the creation of Sparkle's own audio CD. Demonstrating specialist equipment that helps peoples' independence, including that of Cathy's Nana, got the children thinking in positive ways to help those less fortunate than themselves.

As well as teaching, Cathy was so driven to supporting the work of charities, particularly one local Charity; Galloways for the Blind, based in Penwortham. Cathy is a wonderful person, an inspiration to so many, whom I admire so much, not just because of her resilience, but for who she is and her 'never give in, never give up' spirit. She still wants not only to fight against the illness, but help support others living with this condition, and ultimately save lives. I'm so proud to call her a friend.

Kevin Lonergan – Sight Loss Advisor at 'Galloways Society for the Blind'

CHAPTER EIGHT: Childhood dreams for ME
"All the world's a stage!" for Cathy.

"To achieve great things, two things are needed: a plan and not quite enough time" – Leonard Bernstein.

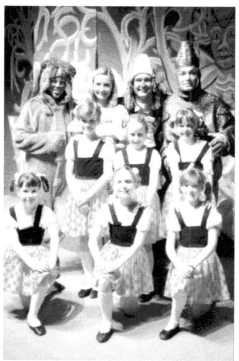

Catherine Vandome age eleven, as a 'Munchkin' in the Ronnie/Trafford Parnell Productions U.K. Tour of 'The Wizard of OZ', with Keith Hopkins as the 'Scarecrow', and fellow munchkins; Helen Latham/Morfitt and Carolyn Bolton/Kidman Beeson, at the Charter Theatre, Preston, in 1985.

Cathy was a happy contented baby, who showed an early talent for performing. Even before her fourth birthday, she loved dressing up and performing in the house and garden.

We enjoyed encouraging Cathy, and her brothers to produce 'shows' during their childhood. On one occasion, a large cardboard box provided the stage for a puppet show. Cathy and her friend Jennifer made tickets, which they insisted were necessary to see the show.

A neighbour popped round to watch and commented on how much she enjoyed sitting in her garden during these productions and listening to Cathy and Jennifer singing.

Cathy held no fears as she grew up and sometimes, she was impulsive in her efforts to achieve what she wanted. Whenever we were out walking near any water, or just paddling, Cathy would always be the one to fall in!

She thrived in a theatre environment and was an excellent dancer with a beautiful singing voice.

Aged nine, Cathy confidently appeared in a school play as 'Mrs. Mopp'.'Throughout her childhood, she had been selected to appear in a number of professional Ballet and Pantomime productions, including playing a Snowflake in 'The Nutcracker and the Mouse King' by The Lewis London Ballet Company and a dancer in Ronnie Trafford/Parnell's Pantomime, 'The Wizard of OZ' with Keith Hopkins.

At the age of thirteen, Cathy was selected to appear as an 'orphan' in the Preston Musical Comedy Society (PMCS), a semi-professional local theatre group, with strong competition from the girls in the Preston area.

I loved being one of the parents, who helped to chaperone the girls during the rehearsals, and I proudly watched her perform.

There was a puppet show included as part of the production, and the girls asked the theatre staff if they could watch it, but had been refused. At the dress rehearsal they were told to remain in their dressing room after leaving the stage and to stay there. They wanted to see the puppets so much that Cathy asked me if it would be possible.

I decided to creep around the back of the theatre with the girls, and gave them instructions to sit on the floor near the exit and to keep completely quiet. They watched the puppet show before excitedly returning to the dressing room, where no-one was any the wiser...until now!

In her professional career, as in her childhood, Cathy enjoyed playing comedy characters and old ladies. A 'proud' parent moment was when we travelled to the Yvonne Arnault Theatre in Guildford in 2000, to see her perform the comical part of 'Grandma Tzeitel' in 'A Fiddler on the Roof' and we hardly recognised her!

Later, we went to the Fortune Theatre in London's West End to watch her sing 'Bill' from 'Showboat' and perform a Lancashire comedy sketch for her Guildford School of Acting (G.S.A.) West End Showcase.

Another memorable time, was visiting Norfolk, to see her playing 'Fairy Sunbeam' in the pantomime 'Sleeping Beauty', for Barrie Stacey Productions, performing once again with Keith Hopkins, as the 'Dame'.

Cathy's determination helped her to succeed, plus her warm heart, caring nature and joy for life.

'All the world's a stage' for Cathy. Happy memories!
Marie Vandome - Author Cathy's Mum

My parents absolutely loved the theatre, and being an attractive young pairing, they actually met each other on the stage, in a local amateur production.

At the opening of Act Four within the play, my mother was directed to sit on my father's knee, wearing just a negligee set, but disappointingly for them both, rehearsals always seemed to end in Act Three!

As neither of them wanted to turn professional, they encouraged their three children, my elder brother, and younger brother, and I, to entertain them with music, singing, dancing and acting, at every given opportunity of the day. We were their court jesters, and the family Vandome costume and props box was overflowing!

I learned from my parents that this 'babysitting strategy' was the best way to entertain children, with the least hands-on childcare duties, in telling us to, "Go and make up a show and come back in an hour and we will watch it!" Years later, with my own children's theatre school, I made a career out of it!

I was a confident, energetic and excitable character. I wasn't afraid of anything and absolutely nothing held me back. The whole world was a stage for me, right from a very young age, and life was for the taking! My family home was my first stage. Our lounge was divided by two crimplene chocolate brown proscenium arch curtains, complete with a 'leg' (a pull string acting as a lever to open and close the curtains).

This was my first experience of the theatrical term, 'break a leg', which actors say to one another before a performance. This is oftentimes misunderstood to mean, 'break a leg' (as in your own leg), but what it actually means is to have such a wonderful performance, with so many encores and curtain calls at the end of the show, that the backstage 'leg of the curtain' rotates so many times it breaks, due to the curtains being repeatedly opened and closed. My elder brother was in charge of this leg.

My mother and father excitedly awaited the theatrical show, seated together on the large chocolate brown lounge settee. Dad puffed on his black pipe, whilst mum cleared her best coffee table out of the way, so that we didn't break it with our 'legs'!

"Please welcome onto the stage… Cathy and David!!" my elder brother announced.

I arrived centre-stage singing, wearing an old white tablecloth on my head, dressed as a bride, and with two front teeth missing, looking more like the bride of Dracula.

Two-year-old David was donned in our mother's favourite curly blonde wig, reluctantly walking behind, sucking his thumb, and holding my train and a large bouquet of plastic flowers. To date, that's the nearest I got to an actual wedding! Singing, dancing and comedy flowed from us all, and with Dad providing the dry-ice smoke from his pipe, unable to see clearly, we almost always ended the show with an accidental injury!

In 1983, aged nine years old, the school headmaster Mr. Fox, cast me as a comedy old lady, 'Mrs Mopp', in the end of school year musical comedy production. This role was a Julie Walter's style of a Mrs. Overall's type of character, and I remember feeling very flattered, because the headmaster told me that I had 'great comic timing' and I was invited to perform this role in the school year above's theatrical production.

Mr. Fox was the first influential person to help guide me into a career on stage as a 'comic entertainer'. I was dressed in a green tabard with a matching headscarf and rollers in my hair, with bright red lipstick drawn larger than my mouth. Holding a large mop, using over exaggerated gesticulations with a broad Lancashire accent, I wouldn't have looked out of place in the TV series, 'Hi de Hi'.

This was the beginning of a career in playing comedy old ladies, and I soon learned that these roles were my favourite, as they always made people laugh. Making people laugh was by far the best feeling in the world. Following this school production, my headmaster recommended that I start to audition for local amateur dramatics societies in Preston, and this prompted my first audition at the age of nine years at The Preston Playhouse Theatre, for a part in that year's Christmas pantomime, The Wizard of Oz.

The Wizard of Oz was being directed by Mrs. Marilyn Brandwood-Spencer, a well-respected local theatrical director and actor, who became a very influential theatrical figure in my future career. I was cast alongside the very talented, Sophie McDonnell, and the equally talented Julie Webster who was playing, the 'Good Fairy'.

The director, Marilyn said that she saw something special in my performance, and she said that she believed in me. Marilyn also told me that, "As I was being cast as a ballerina 'Munchkin', singing and dancing to 'the lullaby league', I was best learning how to dance, as my toes in my step kicks were anything but pointed!"

I admired Marilyn, as she always told the truth, in order to encourage performers and prepare them for the world of professional theatre. I took her advice, and I immediately started ballet and modern dance classes at the 'Barbara Saunders Jones Dance School' in Preston.

Barbara Saunders Jones was an incredibly hard working, eloquent, disciplined and influential dance teacher, who was instrumental in my professional career, as she laid the foundations of the professional dancer I became.

Mrs. Jones was also very honest, and she once said to my mother, "Cathy may not be the best, but she certainly tries the hardest."

I was so passionate about ballet dancing that at the age of thirteen, Mrs. Jones sent me to audition to be a ballerina in a professional touring production of, 'The Nutcracker and The Mouse King' with 'The Lewis London Ballet Company', at The Charter Theatre in Preston.

"When I sent you to an audition for a professional ballet dance company, then I obviously saw something very special in you, or I wouldn't have sent you."
Barbara Saunders Jones - Dance Teacher at the Barbara Saunders Jones Dance School and Awarded 'Life Member of The Royal Academy of Dance' (RAD). (Recently deceased).

I walked nervously with feet turned out, onto The Charter Theatre stage, dressed in a black leotard, pink ballet tights and pink satin ballet shoes, which were laced at the ankle with pink ribbons, and sprayed with hairspray to glue them tight.

My hair was tied tightly back into a ballet bun, also glued with hairspray, and my mother had accessorised by clipping a huge white 1980's fashion bow onto my head. I was surrounded by a sea of hundreds of aspiring ballerinas from all over the Northwest of England, all dressed almost identically. Some diva mothers were following their children onto the stage, frantically spraying hairspray all over their child in a last-minute bid to make them as toxic as they were!

I could feel the tension in what little air was left! This didn't feel like my past experiences of fun amateur auditions, this looked like a very serious competition, and it was to be my first ever professional audition.

Downstage centre, the leading choreographer and ballet dancers introduced themselves and explained that the turnout today was a far larger number than they had expected.

Overly keen mothers were then sternly advised to, "Please leave the stage in order for the audition to commence!" I have no doubt that some of them would have auditioned themselves given half a chance!

I looked around me and I smiled at a couple of dancers I knew. I would normally have been chatting and laughing… but this was appearing to be no laughing matter! This was very serious indeed.

Dancers surrounding me were stretching their legs and performing demi plies and extending their limbs high in the air, whilst looking down their noses at me. That wasn't hard to do, as I was tiny in stature, but they were behaving like peacocks. I learned on this day, that many dancers behave this way to see off the competition, so in return I smiled and pulled my leotard out of my bum!

The choreographer began teaching everyone the dance routine as best she could, with a blanket of so many young dancers before her; we were all falling over each other into the wings.

The choreographer said that the Ballet Company were only looking for 'six' ballerinas to play 'Snowflakes' in the main segment of 'The Nutcracker and the Mouse King', and after this they were going to choose mice and toy soldiers and other characters within the Ballet.

I didn't like this feeling. My immediate thought was that I have absolutely no chance of getting through, everyone is far prettier and slimmer and more talented than me. Why am I even here?

The music began, and adrenaline started to surge through my body, a combination of excitement and fear. I held in my stomach tightly and barely breathing, I performed the ballet routine to the best of my ability, taking turns with the other girls to join the front line of the audition process, to be judged.

The choreographer stopped the music and looked out at the overspilling stage of young hopeful ballerinas before her, and began the selection process.

Despite being aged thirteen, I looked aged nine, and I was positioned centre stage behind much younger girls than me, all towering above me on either side, and blocking my vision or any chances of my being seen.

The first two ballerinas out of six were selected from the crowd.

"We are looking for a ballet dancer who is wearing a large white bow in her hair," came the voice. Immediately, every expectant girl with any kind of white ribbon or handkerchief they could find, placed it on their head, and one by one, confidently stepped forward to accept their reward.

One by one, I heard sarcastically, "No! No! No! Not you dear!"

Suddenly, I felt a shove from behind me, and a kind dancer shouted out, "What about her, she was wearing a large white bow in her hair, but it's fallen out!"

Embarrassed, I stood still holding my large white bow in my open palm, as the parting of the waves happened and girls stepped aside, so that I could be seen.

"Yes! Yes! It's you girl. It's definitely you! Step forward and join the other Snowflakes downstage!"

I couldn't believe my luck! I still thought they had probably mixed me up with a much better dancer than me, but they seemed convinced that I was 'Snowflake' number three.

'The Lewis London Ballet Company' went on to cast the remaining dancers, and I should have been excited, but I simply froze in shock and disbelief at what had just happened. I was fully prepared at any time for them to confirm their selection process error!

During the full week's run of 'The Nutcracker and The Mouse King', some of the professional dancers kindly told me that I had a natural flair for ballet, alongside a tiny frame, and discussions over my future career were raised. Following my luck in getting into 'The Lewis London Ballet Company' production, it was recommended by the ballerinas, and my dance teacher Barbara Saunders Jones, that I go to a ballet school to train to become a professional ballerina.

I really wanted to go, but I was advised that it would disrupt my schooling, and be a huge financial expense. I was told that, like all aspiring ballerinas, I would most likely only perform in the 'corps de ballet.'

I would not be able pursue other passionate art forms, which I enjoyed equally, like drama and singing, and I certainly wouldn't be allowed to do any comedy! My heart was in musical theatre, a hybrid of all three disciplines, and so we decided I would audition for drama schools when I was older. Also, my parents felt that aged thirteen was too young to be moving out of my family home and starting a professional career in the arts, and that my education was important too.

I continued performing in many local theatre productions both professional and amateur shows, including becoming a member of 'Preston Musical Comedy Society' (P.M.C.S.), performing in Musical Theatre productions, as well as Shakespeare plays, Pantomime's, Ballet's, Youth Theatre productions, and numerous dance shows. I was lucky enough to be chosen to perform as a 'Munchkin' at The Charter Theatre, Preston, in Trafford/Parnell Productions UK Tour of 'The Wizard of Oz'. This was a professional pantomime, and I was cast alongside my talented musical theatre friends, Helen Latham/Morfitt and Carolyn Bolton/Kidman Beeson.

The very talented, Keith Hopkins was playing the scarecrow, and in years to come, I would be both amazed and grateful to have the opportunity once more, to share the stage with him.

As a thirteen-year-old teenager, I auditioned for Preston Musical Comedy Society, and I was cast as one of the child 'orphans', in the production of 'Annie' at The Charter Theatre, Preston. I looked the same age as the other younger orphans, who were aged nine and up, and I was delighted to be joined by my talented friends, Helen Latham/Morfitt, playing the lead role of 'Annie', along with fellow orphans, Alison Carthy, Carolyn Bolton/Kidman Beeson, Karen Holmes, Marli Harwood (Marilena Buck), Katy Lanson and other very talented young girls.

This production of 'Annie' was as good as any professional musical production, and I was once again honoured to be joined by Julie Webster, who this time was terrifyingly talented as Miss Hannigan.

The choreographer was an old-school professional, and she was equally terrifying, but her dance routines were incredible, and she achieved perfect, slick and professional results.

During the evening's dress rehearsal, I was on stage, sharing an orphanage bed with Alison and Carolyn, when the choreographer bellowed, "If any of you orphans don't hit your mark with your scrubbing brushes and buckets downstage by the second beat of the music for, 'It's a hard knock life', then you won't be allowed in the number!"

As a perfectionist, and afraid of authority figures, I took her warning very seriously. As soon as the musical introduction began, I leapt out of our wooden bed faster than any other child, straight into my silver metal bucket by my bed, and I got my large black boot stuck inside it.

Determined not to let anybody down, I dragged that bucket on one leg downstage, and my goodness I hit my mark with my old scrubbing brush in hand, banging it on the floor on the second beat of the music, as per her instruction!

It was the first time the choreographer turned a little shade of red, and she respectfully allowed me a moment to remove the bucket from my foot, of which I needed help from fellow orphans, before continuing with the number. That night I came very close to kicking the bucket!

We all thoroughly enjoyed this experience, and inspired by this P.M.C.S. production, many of us went on to perform in the entertainment industry professionally. Here, within the cast, I met another inspirational actor and mentor Eddie Regan, admired by all within the heart of my hometown of Preston. Eddie shared valuable stage performance words of wisdom with me, and I was honoured to be a part of this Society, and I remain so.

"I have been involved with Preston Musical Comedy Society for 63 years and known Cathy for many years. I have such fond memories of our time together, in

many shows. I remember her boundless energy and enthusiasm and obvious great talent.x"
Eddie Regan – Actor and Vocalist, Preston Musical Comedy Society

A year later, at aged fourteen, I was cast as 'Joseph' in, 'Joseph and the Amazing Technicolour Dreamcoat.' I was absolutely shocked to be chosen to play this lead role, and I didn't believe I was worthy of it.

My very talented acting mentor, Carol Buckley was an inspiration to me, she believed in me and encouraged me to try to have confidence in myself throughout this production. I performed alongside a wonderful cast, including my talented childhood friend, Jennifer Woodburn, as one of the brothers, and we were joined by our virtuoso friend, Stephen Pettinger, who constantly made me laugh backstage to try to calm my nerves, as he seamlessly played a truly captivating 'Narrator.'

In 1990, at age sixteen, I was blessed to be cast as, 'Princess Melanie' opposite the talented Alison Carthy as my Prince, in the pantomime, 'Humpty Dumpty', and we shared the stage with the very naturally gifted, Dermot Canavan, at The Preston Playhouse. Dermott rightfully became a professional performer, and his comic timing playing alongside me as a comedy henchman, was impeccable. I learned a great deal about comic timing from his performances, and we shared the inability to stop laughing, resulting in a great deal of 'corpsing' on stage.

The same year, I was lucky enough to be chosen once again to perform with 'The Lewis London Ballet Company', in the Ballet production of 'Alice in Wonderland' at The Charter Theatre, Preston. I was cast as, 'The Queen of Spade's Ballet Dancer Playing Card'. The incredible life-long friendships, which I was blessed to make, alongside the professional training, and confidence building in multiple disciplines, which all stemmed from performing on stage in my youth, would serve to last a lifetime, and this is why the world of entertainment is so valuable to the youngsters of today. The world of theatre was pure joy and fast becoming my whole world. The adrenaline high was addictive.

I first met my friend Cathy around 1981, as we were both enthusiastic members of our local dance school, taking ballet, tap and modern dance classes in a church hall in Fulwood, Preston.

Living no more than five minutes from her, we were also both part of the Catholic community, going to the same church, at the painfully early 8.30am Sunday service, sweetened by the Church Breakfast that followed in the hall!

Dance classes led to many chances to perform in shows at local theatres: munchkins together in 'The Wizard of OZ'; villagers in pantomimes, and most memorable personally, 'orphans', where I played 'Annie' in the Preston Musical Comedy Society's, 'Annie' which changed my life and led me to acting as my future profession.

As high energy as me, always bounding around, Cathy became a great playmate, though I also remember many frustrating bouts of tonsillitis and other infections that she suffered, when the showbiz had to pause.

It was the connecting moments that fed our giggly friendship - the routines carefully choreographed in theatre dressing rooms and girly bedrooms to 'Wham', the performances of these to parents forced to sit on sofas and be an adoring audience, the taking over of the church choir and attempts at high harmonies at 8.30am, the ridiculous, infectiously funny drama sketches concocted that no one else would 'get' and a lot of silliness in general!

A loyal friend, Cathy was and is always positive, and happy to poke fun at herself.

Teenage years beckoned, boys entered the mix, bringing drama good and bad, and we sang and danced our way through it. As Cathy headed off to university for the first time to pursue her dream of a performing career, I was wedged in the back seat of her parents' car, between boxes and cases, and saw some of her freshers' week with her, (an exciting new world, as I was two school years' younger).

We both enjoyed careers in entertainment, taking us all over the world, and at my wedding in 2004, Cathy was first up on the dance floor, boogying with my dad! Ten years later, events took a sadder turn when I heard she had collapsed with ME, which I knew little about.

In 2020, for my dad's funeral, Cathy, with the help of her lovely man, Mark, and less lovely walking stick, made it to the church, giving me her condolences with an unsteady stance, at the same steps we used to bound down giggling!

Trips from my southern life back home to my mum have to include a visit to Cathy's whenever possible, where she's always full of laughter and fun, though we can't do 'Wham' routines now as she's often tired.

I now know more about ME, and Dr Perrin and his treatments, and I hope this leads to her recovery one day, her return to a stage near you!

Resilient, patient and eternally good-humoured, Cathy deserves to go onwards and upwards as ME slowly becomes less misunderstood, and Dr Perrin continues to help progress!

Helen Morfitt – Actress and Starlight Kids Musical Theatre Owner

CHAPTER NINE: Educating ME
Big School! – Well, every school was big to me!

"The human body is the only machine for which there are no spare parts." – Hermann Biggs.

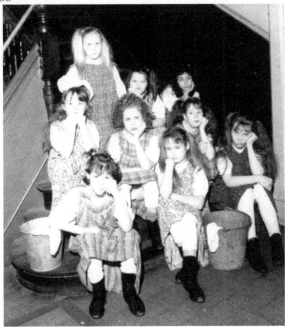

Catherine Vandome age thirteen, as an 'Orphan' in the Preston Musical Comedy Production of 'Annie', with **Helen Latham/Morfitt as 'Annie'**, along with fellow orphans; **Alison Carthy, Carolyn Bolton/Kidman Beeson, Karen Holmes, Marli Harwood (Marilena Buck) and Katy Lanson**, at the Charter Theatre, Preston, in 1987.

My best friend Cathy. My first memory of Cathy was meeting her at Barbara Saunders Jones' Dance school. I was in the next class and I watched her dancing through the window and was surprised at her high level of mobility and arch in her spine, as she was performing a flat back stretch. I looked in on one huge smile! I knew then, aged thirteen, that we were going to be mates for life!

We walked to school together and sometimes we took our bikes with a basket on the front...we didn't care! I even asked for a reflective stripe for Christmas like Cathy's! We never rode them, we just walked and chatted. Not everyone appreciated this, as we did take up the entire pavement.

There was 'never' a dull moment with Cathy. We laughed and laughed until we were exhausted. We were always singing and dancing and Cathy also played the organ. My favourite song that she sang was 'Paper moon', and my favourite organ piece she played was 'Perfidia' and together we choreographed a lovely dance routine on my mum and dad's patio to The Brits tape!

We performed at the Preston Playhouse Theatre together in the Christmas pantomime 'Aladdin', which was lots of fun.

Cathy is a beautiful soul, who would never dream of hurting anybody. A fragile heart growing up and always saw the best in people. We were bullied by some girls on the way to and from school. Every morning there was a comment and then a punch in the face for Cathy!

I remember Cathy had constant tonsillitis and very fragile health and was always on antibiotics. She had fainting episodes, nose bleeds, hay fever, thrush and very heavy periods with pain so bad she often had to go home from school!

As we grew up Cathys health affected both of us, as Cathy was the life and soul of the party and I hated it when she was ill and couldn't come out! I used to pray the evening before that she would recover in time, but she barely did, which was sad.

Cathy is trusting, loyal and such a bloody good laugh. Entertainment all the way with V - my nickname for her. Cathy was first up…upside down on our Barfly at The Preston Guild 1992. She won the family party game of picking up a cereal box with your teeth…Cathy was so flexible she was in the splits within a second!

Cathy and I danced on ITV's 'The Hitman and Her', in Tokyo Joe's Night-club in Preston with Pete Waterman and Michaela Strachan, shaking our heads to, 'Felix don't you want me?' and we were on stage with The Drifters.

We went on our first holiday together to Ibiza and by the end of the week we were performing singing and dancing on stage with the hotel entertainers! We worked together at Broughton Park Hotel. Cathy transferred from Barton Grange Hotel, as I had to have her by my side!

We enjoyed bat and ball and picnics in the park and watching lots of comedies and horror films together. Fun - Fun - Fun!

I went with Cathy to her first drama school audition on the train, and I can remember her piece ended with "like granite!"

Years later, I was in the audience when Cathy was on stage as the presenter for L'Oreal, for a Boots corporate event. So many fantastic memories and not one bad experience! How many people can say that about their best friend growing up. Cathy you were my childhood and I love you xxxx.

Louisa Cornall – Customer Services Advisor - Financial Services

It was September 1985 and my first day of high school. I felt so grown up, as I walked up the main school pathway and through the big, iron, school gates of St. Cuthbert Mayne high school, now Our Lady's Catholic high school. I wore a crisp, freshly ironed maroon school uniform, with a starched white shirt, and matching knee length white socks. My maroon under-the-knee pencil skirt was rolled up three times at the waist, to avoid me tripping over it, and yet was still full length on me. My oversized maroon V-necked jumper had my sleeves turned up twice on my doll sized arms, to provide growing room which was never needed!

I may have felt grown up, but I certainly looked anything but!

I was tiny in stature, and as I passed through the school gates, a number of older children were pointing and laughing at me. I didn't mind this happening on stage, but not as I walked into big school...and to me this was indeed big school! I overheard one girl laughing, saying, "Look at the size of her!"

She was right. I was one of the smallest in my year group, and remained so. This provided bullies with instant material, not original, but then bullies never are. Being so short hugely knocked my confidence, and so I knew that I had to try extra hard to try and be funny, so that I could fit in, and be liked.

My strict catholic high school headmaster entered the large school assembly hall, donned in a black cap and gown, which billowed and eerily followed behind him down every corridor, long after he had disappeared from sight. His very presence convinced me that death is nigh and his job was to command the utmost of respect and instil fear into every single pupil by highlighting that, "If the school rules are broken there will be consequences!"

My newly formed, inquisitive first-year group were shown around the entire school grounds, and I remember thinking that this was the biggest school I had ever been in, and that I would surely get lost changing classes. I felt like 'Alice in Wonderland'.

We were firmly directed to, "Always walk on the right hand side of the corridor to avoid colliding with pupils passing on the left". This was surely a flawless system? Being obedient and terrified of authority, I took my corridor directions a bit too literally. One morning, as I was walking to assembly on the right-hand side of the corridor, I found that I was so far over to the right that... Bang! I walked straight between the eyes into the corner of a large picture frame hanging on the wall.

I went dizzy and fell faint, and as my legs went from under me, a teacher passing by caught me and came to my aid.

The teacher took me straight to the school office for a glass of water.

I thanked her, and I told her that I was absolutely fine, as I didn't want to be late for class, but I hadn't realised that the bang to the centre of my forehead was so strong, that I had blood dripping down my face. The teacher asked me how I had hit my head, not believing that I had walked into a picture frame on the wall. Believing instead that I had been punched, she laughed in disbelief saying that, "It was physically impossible for me to bang my head on a picture frame in the school corridor, as they were hanging at far too low a level."

And I guess that explains just how short I was. It would have been far less humiliating to agree with her. I was kept in the office for a long while, as my head wouldn't stop bleeding...and she couldn't stop laughing!

Throughout my first year at high school, my passions for Drama, English, Music, Arts and Sports continued, and subjects like Maths, Geography and History were endured. Life was for the taking. I would look at my school time table and feel excited each day when my favourite subjects were on that day's school planner. I didn't like sitting still. I was very excitable, and I always had a project on the go. I would daydream in lessons that were of no interest to me.

I was disappointed in the summer months to be absolutely streaming sneezing, with red runny eyes, from a diagnosis of family hay fever, so bad that I was at times not allowed out onto the playing fields with the other children.

One afternoon, during the science class, on the teacher's instruction, the whole class excitedly lined up to go outside to enjoy looking at the school's 'nature surrounds', studying trees, plants, and leaves. What a joy to get out of a hot science room, and out into nature, but due to the level of my health condition, I was left behind alone, using my Beconase nasal spray and Otrivine eye drops, and told to "read a science book about leaves instead." Sat alone in silence, I leafed through the pages.

This was reminiscent of my young childhood, where I had to have private reading lessons alone for fear of particular stimuli, however in this case I wasn't afraid of leaves, but I was undoubtedly afraid of missing out on having any fun!

I knew from a young age, that all I wanted to do was spend the whole of my life on stage entertaining, so I couldn't see the point in learning Pythagoras' theorem. My drama teacher, Mrs Connor, quickly spotted my passion for drama, and kindly told me that she thought I had a great deal of talent for this subject. She encouraged me throughout my high school years to focus on this subject, which I did, both inside and outside of school.

Mrs Connor chose my friend Jennifer Woodburn and I, to perform a theatre piece to the entire school year group assembly. I was playing the role of 'Helen Keller' and Jennifer was playing 'Helen's guardian'.

It was a very challenging piece, with the character of Helen being deaf, dumb and mute. The rehearsals involved Jennifer's character attempting to feed me with a large spoon, with my character spitting the food out in her face, before leaping full length down the table, and knocking everything over.

During rehearsals and being young teenagers, watching the rice pudding I had just spat at Jennifer, dripping slowly down her face, made me corpse, and we both started belly laughing.

Mrs Connor bellowed, "If you laugh…you'll get graded an E for your GCSE!" We both agreed from now on, not to make any eye contact, for fear of giggling. Mrs Connor also threatened me with, "Cathy, if you play another old lady, you will get an E!" This instruction I ignored, and I ended up making a professional career out of it!

During my second year of high school, now aged thirteen, my best friend Louisa and I were walking to school, when two girls from another High School were passing us on the street. One of the girls suddenly punched my friend in the mouth and split her lip. The girl warned me, "I'm coming back for you tomorrow, so watch out!"

True to her word, the following morning she assaulted me, and punched me so hard in the face that she broke my nose. The blow split the bridge of my nose and splatted blood all over her and me. There was so much blood that she looked as shocked as I was, as she and her friend scurried away. Instead of thinking about the pain, all I could think was, 'Thank goodness my school uniform is maroon to hide all the blood!'

The following day Louisa's father, John Cornall, and my mother joined us on the way to school to warn off these bullies. John pretended to be a police man, and my mother took her prior acting training very seriously, and brought a prop notepad and pen, playing the part of a local journalist.

After John gave the two girls "a good telling off", my mother's role was silent but deadly, as she balanced her glasses on the bridge of her nose, and frantically scribbled into her notepad, before using her disposable camera skills to capture the moment. These bullies never bothered us again.

During my first year of high school, all the students were given a compulsory medical check and this included checking the spine for any potential structural abnormalities. The rotund school nurse stood at my side, and asked me to lean forwards from the waist. Compliantly, I placed my hands and my elbows flat on the floor in front of me. The nurse looked down at me in complete shock.

"This is the first time I have seen anyone this flexible!" she exclaimed.

I gleefully awaited a round of applause and a circular, red lolly for my magic trick. No response.

Instead, like a performing monkey, the nurse asked me to perform more unrewarded tricks. Next, I was asked to stand with my feet together as instructed, whilst she pointed out that I had very sway back legs, my knee joints extending beyond the normal range, causing a gap inside my legs when my feet were closed together.

"My nickname is banana legs!" I joked. No laugh, but then it was a tough crowd! The nurse was increasingly interested in my 'exterior', and I wondered how much money I would make for her in the circus?

I was then asked to walk in a straight line.

"Your hyper-mobile joints are causing fallen arches, where the arches of your feet are rolling inwards, when positioned flat on the floor," the nurse explained.

Judging by her expression, none of these diagnoses were deemed positive and keeping me out of the circus. The nurse finally examined my whole frame.

"All your joints are hyper mobile and your spine and shoulders are very rounded and curved. I want you to see your doctor about this, as this will put enormous strain on your joints as you grow, and likely cause you pain. You must learn to stand with a straight back and hold your shoulders back," she instructed.

I agreed that I would do anything to make myself look taller!

The doctor instructed me to wear a pair of brown rubber shoe insoles. "You must wear them inside your shoes and trainers, at all times, to help support your fallen arches."

The doctor then demonstrated a set of exercises to practise at home three times a day, which were best demonstrated by Barbara Windsor in the classic comedy film, "Carry on Camping".

"Oh good," my mother excitedly replied in front of the doctor, emphasising the dual benefits of the exercises… "I must, I must, improve my bust! This will help you to develop a bust at the same time!"

Pin drop…

Her words were comically expressed in that all-too-familiar embarrassing mother tone, as I hung my head on my hyper-mobile neck in shame.

Following this, I only went bra shopping with my mother once.

"She doesn't need one yet, but all her friends are wearing them…" I was twenty-four!

My mother had her values. By knowing my extensive medical history, and allergic reactions to medications, she thankfully contacted my high school to tell them that I had already had German Measles, and I wouldn't be needing the MMR Vaccine. My mother was told by the school medical board, "It is not possible for your daughter to have already had German measles before the age of twelve years. She will be taking that vaccine unless you can provide full medical evidence of this."

My mother fought hard to get a signed letter from my GP confirming my diagnosis of German Measles at the age three, which only just arrived in time before the vaccine would have been administered.

Later on, now aged thirteen, the B.C.G. booster vaccine was about to be administered in school. All students were to have a 'six needles' test prior to the vaccine being given, for safety.

I returned to class with a red swollen left arm, and I was told that I had failed my test dose of the B.C.G. vaccination, (Booster) and I would not be able to take it, due to having a severe allergic reaction.

All my friends returned to class wearing huge smiles on their faces and gloating at the pain they had overcome, in order to have a huge raised lump on their upper left arm, which remained for years, like a high school stamp seal of approval. As a perfectionist, I wanted to be like everyone else and fit in, but unable to have my stamp and with hyper mobile joints, I began packing my bag for the travelling circus.

"You girl! Come to the front of the assembly!" The headmaster angrily pointed at me.

I nervously walked forward to the front of my form group, fully aware of why I was being told off.

"I have permission from my drama teacher, Mrs Connor for this hairstyle." I gently defended myself.

I was playing the role of 'Puck', in 'A Midsummer Night's Dream' at The Preston Playhouse, and I was permitted for the week of 'show run', to wear my hair in a large plait interwoven with pipe cleaners, standing vertically upwards, central to my head. Mrs Connor had forgotten to tell the Headmaster, and this was the only time she got herself into trouble. Post public humiliation, I was directed back in line, as I silently gave her an 'E' for 'competence!'

My passion for all sports continued throughout high school, and despite being one of the smallest girls in my year, my competitive spirit in the face of my 'height adversity', landed me the positions of 'goal shooter' in netball, front runner in relay races, and surprisingly, in Fourth Year (now Year 10) I somehow won the Girls' Long Jump. I was laughed at for this achievement, by members of my own winning form group...but I was used to it by now, and as always, I didn't stand up for myself, for there was no point standing up, as it didn't make me any taller!

In my life so far, I had been a number of mythical beings: a Goblin, a Brownie, and an Elf (Puck) and to be fair, if I saw a 'small industrious fairy' winning school prizes meant for the adult kingdom, I too, may have been a tad disappointed.

I soon started having private table tennis lessons with a local club coach, who was keen to enter me into competitions at the age of fourteen, in spite of having the stature of a ten-year-old. We were both surprised that I could actually see over the edge of the table to play. Used to practising on our home table tennis table in the garage with my father, who played properly against my elder brother, as they both had a gift for this sport, I really enjoyed these lessons.

However, with being my father's only daughter, he dropped his game level at first. Then as time passed, and I saw him sweating and missing my fast forehand swing shots by darting into the lawnmower, I realised that he was now playing properly!

I stood ready for the table tennis competition to begin, bat poised in my right hand, as three men in their twenties and thirties lined up looking embarrassed to have to compete against a little girl in an adult table tennis competition. The first man was a little too certain of his predicted outcome, and I was overjoyed to beat him, with my talented coach, Bill laughing with joy and no doubt surprise.

The first fast win caused the remaining two men to focus much harder, and like my father had learned to do...play properly!

The second and third players beat me only just, by the game's designated two points, and all three men shook my hand afterwards.

The poor, embarrassed first player was about to join them in a post competition pint, and quite likely become the evening's laughing stock, as he'd assumed I would be.

"Get Cathy! Hit her with your hockey stick and get her out of the game!"

I am running at fast speed across the grey outdoor gravel stone, hockey pitch, weaving and darting the challenging opponents, when I hear these words seconds before ...

THWACK!

I am struck hard on my right hand by a large wooden hockey stick. The shock bringing me to a standstill, and silencing me in fear. I drop my hockey stick and grab my hand in pain. The kindly sports teacher immediately comes to my aid, and I am sent inside and advised to go to hospital.

"You have a broken thumb," the doctor explains, pointing at my X-ray. "Considering the black and blue injury, it is only a slight break, but you must wear this plaster cast for six weeks and a sling to hold the weight of it."

I was a school prefect, and as I stood directing students out into the yard at break time, everyone laughed and gave me a 'thumbs up' response to my 'thumbs up' plaster cast. I was lucky it was my thumb and not the middle finger.

I had just been cast as Romeo's footman, 'Balthazar', in a production of 'Romeo and Juliet' at The Charter Theatre, Preston, alongside my talented friend Melanie Ash, who went on to become a professional in the industry. All my fellow actors, laughingly questioned the authenticity of a plaster cast in this time period? Climbing the scaffolded staging with one arm was a challenge, but as always…the show must go on.

Later that year, I was on my way home from school, and after being spat on from behind, I heard a voice shout, "Punch her in the head and take her down!"

Before I had any time to react, a girl at least twice my size, punched me very hard in the right side of my head, knocking my jaw and ear which I could hear ringing, and I fell to the pavement with a thud, momentarily out cold.

My mother had taught me not to fight back and to always walk away from confrontation. I think her advice was likely based on the odds being heavily stacked against my winning any fight, as I was built like Dobby the House Elf.

Dazed, I slowly stood up, holding my head in defence, and ran straight forwards into the road, before the blurred pavement ahead came into sight.

I then ran all the way home like an Olympic athlete. I ran the way I had done as a four-year-old goblin in primary school, only that was for laughs, whilst this was to save myself!

I thankfully graduated high school in July 1989, with all my G.C.S.E.'s, and despite my acting examination piece being a 'comedy old lady', Mrs Connor awarded me with an 'A' for Drama.

I was administered a final dose of Tetanus and Polio.

By the time I graduated, I had endured a bang to the front of my head, a break to the bridge of my nose, a broken thumb, a diagnosis of Extreme Hypermobility, and a blow to the right side of my head. I can confidently say that I went to the school of hard knocks!

My metaphor for life became Chumbawumba's "I get knocked down, but I get up again."

The first time I saw Cathy was in a production of 'A Midsummer Night's Dream' at the Preston Playhouse. She was about fourteen years old and playing the part of 'Puck' alongside some of the more mature stalwarts of the theatre group.

Confident and full of energy, Cathy had no trouble with the text and brought the role to life, lighting up the stage with every scene she was in. I became a fan immediately.

A year later, and I found myself cast in my first pantomime, 'Humpty Dumpty', again at the Preston Playhouse. I was one of the comedy henchmen, and Cathy was 'Principal Girl'. It was obvious from day one of rehearsal that this Princess was not going to be your usual helpless maiden.

Cathy showed that she was not only a terrific actor, performer, dancer and singer, everything you need in a Pantomime Princess, but she also had a great sense of humour, and was a natural when it came to the comedy, happily being the foil to many of my lines and ad libs and we worked well as a team when we weren't corpsing on stage.

I remained at the Playhouse for a few more years whilst Cathy went off to train as an actor. I would always love hearing about how she was getting on, where she was performing and what she was doing.

Always a bundle of life and energy, it was a given that Cathy would succeed in whatever she put her mind too.

Fast forward a few years, and it was my turn to go professional, and I remember seeing Cathy after one particular performance. I was in the Original London Cast of 'Hairspray' at the time, sharing the stage with Mr. Michael Ball, and having the time of my life. Seeing Cathy after one of the shows was a real bonus. Always so positive, bubbly and as ever, full of life. All that was to change though, quite drastically.

Over the years since she fell ill and was diagnosed with ME, I've seen Cathy going from someone full of energy and positivity to the complete opposite, and someone who had no sign of any improvement.

I'm pleased to say that this is changing, for the better and I look forward to the day where I can stand on stage with Cathy again, back where she belongs.

Dermot Canavan - West End Theatre Actor

CHAPTER TEN: Growing pains for ME
Tiresome Teens!

"Fatigue is the best pillow" - Benjamin Franklin.

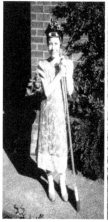
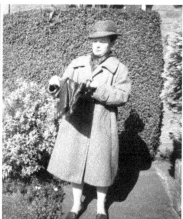

Catherine Vandome age nine, as 'Mrs Mopp' in a Musical Comedy production at Our Lady and St. Edwards Primary School, in 1984.

Catherine Vandome age seventeen, as 'Woman' in Harold Pinter's 'Request Stop', at Preston College, in the 'A' Level Theatre Studies examination, in 1992.

Sitting down to write something for Cathy's forthcoming book, I closed my eyes to see what image would come into my mind. There were two images that immediately sprung to mind...

The first one was of Cathy playing 'Joseph' in The Junior Hall Players production of 'Joseph and the Amazing Technicolour Dreamcoat' at the age of fourteen. Cathy is standing in the middle of the stage wearing her very splendid finale coat. She gave a phenomenal performance, at a very tender age, and was one of those talented young people who could not only sing, but could also act and dance.

The second image that came into my mind, was of Cathy at the age of seventeen or eighteen playing the part of 'Woman' in Harold Pinter's 'Request Stop'.

This image really makes me smile. Cathy was particularly good at playing old ladies (even as a teenager) especially those in the comedy genre, and I think part of this was due to her fabulous comic timing.

Another image that springs to mind is Cathy playing 'Susan' in 'Our Day Out' by Willie Russell. Cathy gave another compelling performance (now in her thirties). Susan was one of the teachers, but as Cathy always looked younger

than her years, she was mistaken for one of the youngsters, by at least one
member of the backstage staff!

I was astounded by the amount of energy that Cathy seemed to possess
in running her very popular summer theatre schools, at which I was often
a guest tutor. She seemed to have a real knack for 'crowd control' and
maintaining the interest of around sixty or so children, whilst making it
look effortless. (I know it wasn't!).

Something else I remember, is when I was rehearsing a Victoria Wood
sketch, about a director giving notes to a bunch of amateurs, and knowing
how good Cathy was at comic timing, I decided to ask her if the script or
my performance could be improved in any way.

I remember having a very good laugh that afternoon as Cathy wrote all sorts of
short lines and explained how she thought they should be delivered. I added these
lines, and it was one of those lines that gained the biggest laugh of the evening.

I really hope that Cathy will eventually make a full recovery and her talent
will once again be used to entertain the people of Preston.

Carol Buckley - LAMDA Drama teacher and Actress.

I started at Preston College in September 1990, taking 'A' Levels in English
Lit/Lang and Theatre Studies, alongside a Performing Arts Diploma, and an
additional G.C.S.E. in Dance. As in my high school G.C.S.E.'s, I worked extremely
hard in all subjects. However, after narrowly missing a grade C in my G.C.S.E.
Maths, I was advised to retake this, to achieve a grade C or above, as I was told
Pythagorus' theorem was important in our society's construct, and I needed to
impress the future Prime Minister!

On 28th November 1991, at 17 years old, I was diagnosed with Glandular
Fever, my GP was involved, and insisted that I had eight weeks complete rest in
bed, housebound. I missed so much college following the months of sickness and
fatigue, that I felt I was forever playing catch up, so I pushed myself ever harder,
to catch up with the rest of the English, Theatre and Dance groups.

Fast asleep, with my head resting atop 'The Colour Purple' English
Literature book, the English teacher politely told the students seated alongside me
at the large rectangular grey table to, "Leave Cathy in peace to sleep."

The extreme fatigue I was experiencing was taking its toll on all my
studies. My flu-like symptoms continued, and I was pleased that I was going to
have access to a large white hanky as a prop for my Theatre Studies practical
examination.

I had thankfully already met my most inspirational drama teacher, Carol
Buckley, at The Hall Players Theatre Group, when I was a young teenager. Carol
not only has an incredible talent for acting, and a meticulous in-depth knowledge
of the performer on stage, but most importantly, she genuinely cares about her
students. Her passion for the theatre and for performing comical old lady
characters, matched my own, and in stark contrast to my high school drama
teacher, Carol positively encouraged me to "Play as many comical old ladies as
you want to!"

Carol taught me about 'character acting' and how to perform the comedy by physically being the character not just playing the role for laughs.

In preparation for my Theatre Studies 'A level' monologue, playing 'Woman' in Harold Pinter's 'Request Stop', Carol gave me extra tuition, outside of college, and she suggested that I observe the mannerisms of an 'old lady' in order to make the characterisation realistic, and for this she set me a very interesting task.

Obviously, I couldn't let the little old lady across the road know that I was actually copying her mannerisms, so under the guise of pretending to interview her for my drama homework about the war, I sat opposite the lady, and asked irrelevant questions, whilst pretending to write down her answers.

I was actually writing down 'how she was sitting', 'the tone of her voice', and 'how she blew her nose and then proceeded to clean her mottled glasses with the same over-sized white hanky!'

This meticulous Stanislavski based observation in creating a character was tutored by Carol, and I followed her teaching to the letter, throughout my own career on stage. Indeed, Carol would lay the foundation of my future career and support my setting up my own drama school, following in her footsteps in years to come.

My Theatre Studies and Performing Arts classes included fellow talented budding actors, and under the tutelage of playwright and very gifted actor, Derek Martin, we performed one of Derek's own plays entitled, 'Our World is in Colour', which was about a group of psychiatric patients living in an institution. To be honest, and I say this jokingly on behalf of the group, we were not straying too far from reality. Or to put it another way, we were surprisingly believable!

The 'A' level theatre performances were to be influenced by the works of any of the three following playwrights and practitioners, whom we had studied during the course: Konstantin Stanislavski, Bertolt Brecht, and Antonin Artaud.

Russian actor, Konstantin Stanslavski's theatre work, is based on naturalism and his legacy was that of 'Stanislavski acting' or 'method acting', his work being founded on the imitation of real life on stage, his method being that both the actor and audience are to fully engage and believe that what they are experiencing is 'real'.

German playwright Bertolt Brecht founded his theatrical method of 'Epic Theatre', an over-expressive theatrical form, including over-gesticulation of the body, where the audience is made constantly aware that they are inside a theatrical space at all times. Brecht wanted to make his audiences think for themselves, and he influenced, amongst others, the work of Playwright and British actor, Stephen Berkoff, in his play 'Metamorphosis'.

Whilst, French actor and director, Antonin Artaud's theatre work, is based on the 'Theatre of the Absurd' and the 'Theatre of Cruelty', a method of theatre influenced by psychologist Sigmund Freud, and his analysis of dreams. Artaud's Theatre, is a therapeutic way of bearing one's soul and releasing desires and emotions into the theatre space, as a form of cathartic release. The belief being that the performers' 'innermost desires' once released, will not need to be released outside of the theatre space, thus healing the individual and consequentially society as a whole.

Antonin Artaud's work influenced actors, and practitioners, including Julian Beck and Judith Malina. Julian Beck was the American actor, who created The Living Theatre, based on the work of Artaud, and is best recognised in Poltergeist 11, as the terrifying villain, Reverend Kane.

I am seated cross legged, within a large circle of my drama peers, inside the cold, dark, blacked-out drama studio space, the cool air rippling the floating black curtains, which are hanging all around the external walls. I am nervously awaiting my turn to perform my Theatre Studies 'A' Level practical examination. After this performance, I am up next.

A student actor eerily enters the circular stage and walks slowly around the centre of the circle looking intimidatingly at each of his audience members.

Suddenly, in an involuntary rage, he shouts out, "I am dying of AIDS and none of you know. I am taking this opportunity to tell you all!" He proceeds to slowly take off all of his clothes, and picks up a large bowl of fruit, and applies it as makeup, all over his face and body, whilst emoting in floods of tears.

There is a breathtaking silence in the studio, the audience are in complete shock, and the examiner promptly leaves the room. The teacher instructs everyone to take a break. I leave the studio and involuntarily cry in shock at what I have just encountered. I believe that our friend is actually dying.

The talented actor had achieved his mission, he had pushed the boundaries of theatre practitioner Antonin Artaud and created a most disturbing piece of 'Theatre of Cruelty', evoking extreme emotional reactions from the audience. Unfortunately for the student, the examiner failed him as he had given 'no prior warning of nudity'. The audience returned, as did the examiner, after much encouragement, and of all things, I had to follow that performance with a comedy sketch of Harold Pinter's 'Request Stop'.

Standing centre stage, next to a mock up bus stop, I am dressed as an old lady, in an oversized, lime green woollen coat, with matching woollen hat and silver rimmed glasses, balanced on the edge of my nose.

"'Beg your pardon, what did you say?" I begin the comic piece, speaking in a broad Lancashire accent. "I know all about it," I continue.

"Standing there, as if butter wouldn't melt in your mouth. Meet you in a dark alley it'd be…another story.''

I remove a large white hanky from my black patent handbag resting over my elbow, and blow my nose loudly and over expressively.

I question what my G.C.S.E. high school drama teacher's reaction would be to my playing yet another old lady!

Fortunately for the examination, I was able to dry my tears, compose myself and learn from this experience the biggest lesson in my theatre career, that no matter what happens, "The show must go on."

It was an exhilarating experience, though highly stressful, and it was made all the better by the previous student apologising and explaining that none of what he had said was true, it was pure Artaud based theatrical spectacle, and for that I personally believed that he should have got top marks! I left the examination, and reflected on how on earth I had managed to make the audience laugh, particularly as I had kept all of my clothes on.

At seventeen years old, I travelled down to London on the train for my first ever drama school audition. I felt very apprehensive about it, and was relieved that my kind-hearted friend, Louisa Cornall had joined me for moral support.

By the end of the train journey, I had recited the entire audition piece to Louisa so many times, that she knew it better than I did! The dramatic piece, which escapes my recollection, ended with the words "...like granite!"

I stayed up all night in a run-down B&B, reciting this darned speech, in front of a broken mirror above a marble sink, unable to sleep, experiencing a mixture of adrenaline and fear.

The drama school specialised solely in theatrical stage acting, and I soon discovered that 'Musical Theatre' was hugely frowned upon here.

"You look like a ballet dancer... not an actor!" The audition panel instantly criticised me as I entered the stage, for unknowingly walking with my feet turned out in first position.

Looking much younger than my years, they continued, "Come back when you have life experience, so that you can truly feel the emotions...This is not musical theatre!"

Despite having had no sleep, I thought I had delivered the line "...like granite" with intense emotion...but I clearly had a lot more to learn! After a couple more failed drama school auditions, I reluctantly resigned myself to going to university.

My practical parents believed that attaining a degree was the most sensible career option and would provide an education and "something to fall back on" should my dreams of working on stage not be realised!

I was grateful that my parents supported my chosen career in the Arts, and I understood their logic behind this decision. However, it wasn't at all what my heart wanted to do.

Every twenty years my hometown of Preston, Lancashire, celebrates all the local trades by having The Preston Guild. Within The Preston Guild are multiple events, including street parties, entertainment, floats and carnival celebrations.

In 1992, I am dancing on top of a moving float and waving a flag high, with my school friends Jennifer Woodburn and Rachel Sharples, celebrating being a part of the local Hall Players Theatre Group. We are costumed all in black, and visible only by a brightly painted face, and mine was a glamorous yolk yellow.

Suddenly, Jennifer drops her flag, and shouts, "Cathy quick jump off the float and get my flag!"

Lost in the deafening music and theatrical surrounds, and not thinking this through, I do exactly what I am instructed to do to save the show! I perform a 'Mission Impossible' running jump off the back of this large moving float...and land sharply on my backside, then into a backward roll...finishing flat on the floor in front of a moving police car, a stunt that Tom Cruise himself would have been proud of. However, I got a very painful back and backside, along with an even more painful 'telling off' from two horrified police officers, who had narrowly missed running me over in their police car.

With no care for myself, I successfully collect Jennifers flag and clamber back up onto the float to gleefully return it to her, and save the show!

During the same year's celebrations, my friend Louisa invited me to her street party and I was dared to demonstrate how to use the hired entertainment outdoor 'Bar Fly'.

After my recent fearless stunt, this was going to be a breeze. With an excited, awaiting street crowd on Barnsfold, in Fulwood, and clad in a 1990's shiny black and blue 'shell-suit style' jumpsuit, with sticky velcro attachments across my back, I fearlessly take a running jump headlong onto the six-foot inflatable wall, and I land perfectly upside down, stuck fast against the 'Bar Fly'...to a big cheer!

When my mother would ask, "If someone told you to jump would you?

My reply was always "Yes, how high?"

In September, aged eighteen years, I was on my way to Manchester Metropolitan University, formally Crewe and Alsager, to study Drama, Dance and Creative Arts. My friend Helen Latham/Morfitt, joined my parents and I, on my first journey to university. It was fortunate that Helen and I were both flexible dancers, as we spent the entire forty-five-minute drive from Preston to Crewe, tightly packed in the back of the car with all the luggage. We were sandwiched precariously between overflowing cardboard boxes, and kitchen utensils, giggling like excitable schoolgirls, as we held onto the door handles for dear life, with every turn in the road!

Sadly, although I made some beautiful friendships here, it was to prove to be a very sickly and unhappy twelve months, after which I was ready to move from the quiet countryside, to the heart of London, to fulfil all my theatre dreams. I was about to start a new BA (Hons) Degree in Dance and Drama, at The Roehampton Institute, University of Surrey.

I first met Cathy in 1990, when we were both sickeningly young, full of hopes and dreams, trying to make our individual dents in the world - via an 'A' level in Theatre Studies at Preston College.

I remember her as fun-loving, and having a lot of laughs, and crucially for me being a bit of a rascal - Cathy was easy target for practical jokes! One thing I remember very clearly, is her introducing me to one of her friends as a 'comedian', which I was pretty thrilled about back then.

I also remember Cathy missing a lot of college the following year, because of Glandular Fever, as it was diagnosed then. I stayed on an extra year at college to retake my Theatre Studies exam and I think Cathy went to uni at Crewe and Alsager. I followed her there a year later, but sadly she left before I got there, so I never saw her after that.

Although years later, I did see her name on a poster at a local pub for a Jessie J Tribute Act - and I thought 'No! It can't be! Can it?' Well life got in the way as it tends to do and I never got the chance to go and find out!

But fast forward thirty years, and thanks to the efforts of Mark Zuckerberg, we've been reunited and I've been delighted to hear she's been writing a book, what a great achievement.

Darren Dutton - Comedy Writer and Social Media Producer

CHAPTER ELEVEN: Perfectionist ME
Another opening of another show!

"Health is not valued till sickness comes" - Thomas Fuller.

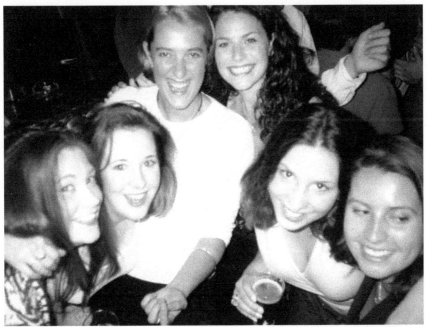

Catherine Vandome with University and fellow entertainer friends Jane Shelley, Paloma Forde, Wendy Pyper, and Joanna Kovats.

Cathy burst into my life quite literally, when I opened my front door to welcome guests to a party my housemates and I were hosting, during my final year at uni.

The theme was 'Camp America' and little did I know that behind the front door was someone who took the meaning of 'Camp' to another level!

Cathy was the shortest of the group of otherwise tall leggy girls in red lycra leotards, recreating 'Baywatch' babes, however it was soon apparent that what she lacked in stature, she made up for in personality and performance. This was a person who loved to entertain, and for the rest of that night Cathy was centre stage in our living room; dancing, singing, joking and noticeably unafraid to send herself up to get a laugh.

The costume choice itself was a comedic decision on her part, (yet I do not believe she realised how fabulous she looked) and reflected the desire to get a laugh, even at her own expense.

The impetus here was making other people happy, and Cathy fed off the energy that bounced back at her in the form of joy, laughter and applause. Her lust for life was infectious and it was obvious to me back then, that this was someone whose career couldn't be anything other than in the entertainment industry!

Despite the confidence displayed on stage, when not in the spotlight, Cathy shows a vulnerable side to herself, and for me this makes her more endearing both on and off the stage.

Since that meeting twenty-five years ago, I have watched Cathy's career grow from strength to strength, as both an all-round entertainer and a teacher.

Even when illness crept in, Cathy would not give up, and I sensed that she felt an obligation to her audience and pupils to carry on, until she physically could not do so anymore. She really does epitomise the age old saying "The show must go on!

Cathy is a lady, who touches people with more joy and laughter than anyone else I know, in addition to being one of the kindest and most supportive and loyal friends. Her determination is an inspiration, and I cannot wait to see Cathy back on stage in whatever reincarnation it will take.

Rolph Patterson - Theatrical Agent, Betty Laine Management (1999-2019)

In September 1993, we enter Froebel college campus through a huge eight-foot wrought iron gate.

"Wow!" my father and I exclaim, as he proudly drives me down a long, winding pathway, towards my new home for the next three years. The Roehampton Institute building in Surrey, and its surrounding scenic grounds, are so grand, that I believe they were used in a number of films, and they ran adjacent to a deer-filled Richmond Park.

There were four quaint cottages on campus, which were situated alongside the large halls of residence, and I was lucky to move into Clarence Lodge Cottage, and live there for the next three years. With a completed first year qualification already under my belt, the university had granted me the option of joining the second year. However, as a perfectionist, I decided to start again in first year, to give myself the best chance of achieving optimum results.

My second attempt at university was to prove highly rewarding and utterly exhilarating, and despite being increasingly unwell, I continued to push through, and thoroughly enjoyed myself, whilst building lifelong friendships.

Now in London, and studying in the place my heart truly wanted to be, I felt exhilarated. At nineteen years old, I was finally fulfilling all my childhood dreams. I was training in Dance and Drama by day, and performing in multiple productions by night, as well as enjoying all the highlights that London had to offer from the West End Theatre shows, to the tourist hot spots, bars, comedy circuits and nightclubs.

I was very happy here. I accepted that I was frequently sick, and this had by now become the norm. I pushed hard against each bout of sickness, so that I could experience it all. I was incredibly hard working and enthusiastic in all things, and I joined numerous evening theatre production groups to keep myself entertained around the clock. As well as performing in musical productions within the university, I also joined 'The Putney Players' where I played 'Amy Spettigue', in a production of 'Charley's Aunt', a farce, by Brandon Thomas.

Playing Amy Spettigue, meant that I had to speak in a R.P. (received pronunciation) accent, and this was challenging, but a great deal of fun. I performed with my talented friend, Sophie Buckman, who was a natural at R.P. and we giggled when I accidentally slipped into a broad Lancashire dialect.

Halfway through one of the performances at The Putney Theatre, I blanked. It was during a comedic scene with a flamboyant character played by a man dressed as a woman, disguised as 'Charley's Aunt', when I completely lost my memory of the script, but I kept going and adlibbed. At the interval, the 'Butler' was blamed for not laying the table quick enough, and to this day the poor man believed it was all his fault. I do hope the Butler can forgive me.

I enjoyed dancing so much, that after a week of dancing in college, I would then go dancing socially with my friends at a variety of central London nightclubs, regularly frequenting 'G.A.Y'., or London's 1970's themed 'Car Wash', as well as a number of local nightclubs, and of course everyone's favourite, the on campus, 'Digby Disco!'

I was so comfortable being lost in the high of the music, that whenever men approached me, I would choreograph a routine and shimmy under their arm to get away, or purposefully start dancing out of time with the music, in the hope that they would leave.

"I love your silver dress," shouted a male voice.

"Thank you!" I replied, whilst spinning away towards my talented dancing friend, Susanne Marston.

"He seems sweet Cathy, have a dance with him," Susanne encouraged me. The man was back.

"You look like a Christmas turkey! I bet you get stuffed tonight!" he hollered.

And with that, Susanne grabbed me away from him, and we made our way back onto the safe platform of the nightclub stage, away from the unoriginal heckler.

My first date at university only served to reaffirm my bad luck with men. The moonlit sky was inviting, and I looked up towards his chiselled handsome face. Our first date had been a success, and he slowly and passionately leaned over from the driver's seat to kiss me. I looked into his deep brown eyes, and turned my head to meet his when...

"OUCH!"

I screamed in his face, as I felt a huge 'BANG' inside my ears, and an overwhelming pain in my jaw. My jaw popped out of line and dislocated. This was immediately followed by another loud 'BANG', as it realigned!

"Arghhh!" I yelled in excruciating pain!

I jumped out of the car, holding my jaw and ran straight into my campus cottage home and didn't look back. As a catholic, it was good to know that I had my own built in self-defence!

I am dancing centre stage atop the highest podium, at my favourite West End nightclub 'G.A.Y.'

Surrounded by incredibly happy men, I feel safe.

Kylie Minogue had just performed on this very podium hours earlier, and with her matching stature, I was now the 'sweaty northern' replacement.

I look like I have just had a fully clothed shower. I am high on the music and the atmosphere. I run my adrenalized, swelled fingers through my long, tangled, drenched brown hair.

Poppas are being passed either side of me.

"What drugs are you on?"

"Sorry?" I reply into the abyss.

As I speak, I am licking black, so called 'waterproof' mascara from the sides of my dry mouth, my plum lipstick and matching lipliner long gone.

"What drugs are you taking to dance like that?" The deep male voice shouts ever louder to be heard above the music. A topless, muscular, bald-headed man pirouettes and extends his large hand out to me, which I take laughing with glee, as I jump into his arms, and he spins me around with ease.

"I don't drink, and I don't take drugs," I reply, sounding like Sandra Dee, showing him my mini, clear blue, plastic bottle of water, as evidence.

"Look at you, you've not stopped dancing all night, I've been watching you. You have the biggest smile. I'm shocked that you are only drinking water!"

"I am high on life!" I shout back laughing. "I love dancing, it's my world."

"Well, you're a great dancer!" He lets go of me and laughs as I thank him, and I double pirouette into the arms of my awaiting dear friend and 'body guard' Rolph Patterson.

Its 4am and we are joined by more of our wonderful friends, including Susanne Marston, Adam Brooks and Sue Coleman, for the finale number of the evening, now very much morning.

"Run for the sun, little one..." 'Bucks Fizz' reverberates through the vast sound system, as dry ice clouds the stage. The group of us start a slow run in unison laughing ever louder with each step forward, as we part the wave of fellow clubbers laughing along with us. The frenetic adrenalized evening ends with "In the land of make believe..." with a 'floorshow spin' from Susanne and I, into our talented friend Rolph's extended open arms, ending in a comedic backbend finale, from all three of us, as laughter is released into the air, when we struggle to retain our balance.

Once outside the club, I crash. My body is freezing cold, and my now, heavy legs struggle to walk. I feel like I am inhaling ice. I push through, and laugh to mask the pain now searing through my body. Rolph notices my teeth chatter and my body shaking uncontrollably, and he generously wraps his jacket around my shoulders. Laughter continues between the group of us, as we recall the long night's entertaining events.

"Same again next week," we all agree, before our long journey home.

Ever caring and considerate, my friends watch me arrive at the gates of my university campus, and as I turn to wave them goodbye, in our shared taxi, they feel assured that I am now home safely. Alone, on an eerily dark and empty street, I turn the eight-foot, wrought-iron, double gate handle, and find that it is locked.

At laser speed, I scan the gate in an upwards motion, and the stark gold rimmed spikes at the top beam at me as a 'warning sign'. I look back at the now ever diminishing taxi, and in a blind panic, I throw myself at the gate, climbing up it in a pair of challenging six-inch, black stiletto heels, and a flowing black dress. In sheer fear, I climb the gate the same way I had done as a one-year-old baby, in achieving the cot gate challenge, but this time without the padded nappy to land on, now grateful for my childhood sports experiences, including high jump, long jump, and running, supporting this Olympic feat.

I look to my right at the campus graveyard, and heavily regret hearing terrifying tales about the nighttime Froebel campus apparition sightings, in addition to hearing that 'The Omen' scene with the priest impaled on a church cross, had apparently been filmed just up the road in Putney, all adding to my adrenal overload. I run so fast in said heels, down the winding road, back home and into the cottage. Hours later, in the splits at 9am, warming up before dance class, I regaled my evenings challenge to my classmates, who were belly laughing and saying that they could not believe that climbing the university, high, wrought-iron gate, was humanly possible.

"Sheer fear can make you achieve anything," I replied. "And believe me, that was sheer fear!"

We all laughed, until the teacher reminded us that, "We don't laugh in Contemporary Dance class".

I thoroughly enjoyed the Drama side of my course, learning more in-depth variants of practitioners' and playwrights' adaptations of stage acting, including giving a Brechtian performance of 'Danton's Death' by the French Renaissance Playwright, Georg Buchner.

This was a most memorable piece, as my talented actress friend Jane Shelley was playing 'Jaques Danton', and I was playing the prostitute, 'Marion'.

We were directed to kiss each other, on stage, and two women kissing in the 1990's, was still considered risqué in performance, and following my recent jaw subluxation, also risky!

Jane and I were used to lining up at the West End Musical 'Grease' for an autograph and a photo with one of the 'T-Birds', and dancing socially together at the 'Digby Disco', yet now here we were about to kiss...and she hadn't even bought me a drink! I was to enact a very moving three-page monologue, the longest I had ever delivered, within the directed Brechtian style of performance. This required that I spoke directly to the audience, whilst costumed all in black with a grey painted face, emulating a chess piece.

"My mother was a good woman. She taught me that chastity was a great virtue..." I began.

In years ahead, this relatively unknown monologue became my main audition piece. I would perform the monologue either seriously as written, or as a comical piece in a broad Lancashire accent. The latter being my preferred choice. I was jokingly re-named 'Miss Catherine Vandermay', just like Hyacinth Bucket as 'Bouquet' in the TV series 'Keeping up Appearances, and this became my stage name. Following my performance, my drama tutor and professional actor, Peter Majer advised that I go to Drama School to get professional training. I am not sure if that *is* a compliment, "Cathy you're very good...so go and get trained!"

I was very flattered that he had said this, as he was currently on screen that year, in 1995, appearing in the James Bond movie 'Golden Eye', playing Valentin's bodyguard, in a scene with Robbie Coltrane.

The following year, in preparation for my finals, I waited outside the 'Dominion Theatre' to meet the cast of the West End musical 'Grease', with my friends, Jane Shelley, Wendy Pyper and Susanne Marston.

"Hi! I'm Catherine Vandermay, and I wondered if I could interview you for my dissertation I am writing about musical theatre," I confidently asked the actor Richard Calkin, playing the lead role of 'Danny.'

I secretly found him very attractive, and my heart raced with excitement, as he accepted my telephone number. I laughed on the tube home that he would never phone me in a million years.

"Ring Ring."

"Cathy! Richard Calkin is on the phone. He's asked to speak to Miss Catherine Vandermay!" squealed my housemate, Lucy Marriott, covering the mouthpiece, as we laughed excitedly, with my thinking that she was joking.

"Hi Richard," I acted outwardly confident, whilst my insides were swirling. "Yes. I can meet you at the stage door on Thursday night and we can go for a coffee, and I will bring my Dictaphone."

"I will bring my Dictaphone!" my words sounding like "I carried a watermelon!", from 'Baby' in the 'Dirty Dancing' movie.

A huge eruption of laughter ensued from my adjoining housemates, all huddled around our hallway landline in disbelief.

Dressed in a black and white business suit and heels, carrying a Dictaphone, I made my way up to the West End Dominion Theatre. Richard welcomed me inside the stage door, and introduced me to Samantha Janus, playing 'Sandy', post matinee performance. He then respectfully, led me to a local theatrical diner, where I felt like Sandy to his Danny, and he kindly offered to buy me a drink.

We sat down opposite each other, and I tried to look professional. Richard broke the ice with his natural wit and jokes, and before long I was recording our interview over the table into my 'high tech' tape recorder Dictaphone. I thanked Richard for his time, and his contribution to my dissertation research, and this momentous occasion served to pave my way of thinking forever, "Don't be afraid to ask for something you want in life. You may not always get it, but your chances are greatly improved by asking."

Following this interview, I contacted Sir Cameron Macintosh's Archives staff, to ask for historical literature, and a week later I was invited to take a look through the archives. I was back in my black and white suit and heels, climbing up large stone steps, weaving through the cast of 'Les Misérables', who were racing downstairs during their matinee performance at the Palace Theatre.

"I dreamed a dream" that day too, and hoped that one day I would have the opportunity to follow in their footsteps.

Back at university, I still had a great deal to learn. As a trained ballet and musical theatre dancer, I found Contemporary dance more challenging to learn.

I was best remembered in my Contemporary dance class, for my choreographed piece entitled 'Balloon Metamorphosis' performed with a number of dance students, including my friend, Sophie Buckman. I say best remembered, because although the dancers performing it were excellent, my piece 'bombed'.

Enjoying pushing the boundaries of performance, I believed that the title of my dance piece, and the long-devoted hours of Laban notation (dance notation) choreography, in passing an invisible balloon to each other, was if nothing else...innovative. However, rather like the physical limitations of my first attempt at choreographing a two-minute contemporary dance piece, by 'hopping on one leg', this too, had its limitations, and was perhaps better suited for the 'French Lecoq school of mime.' The audience laughed.

Not the response I had expected, and I was poorly graded for my efforts, but another sign that I was better suited to comedy. I thought if I am going to get laughed at when I'm trying to be serious, then being funny will be a breeze!

Unlike Mathematics, where the answers are clearly either right or wrong, creative arts subjects are down to the individual's perspective of what is deemed to be credible, or otherwise, and although very funny, my invisible balloons were deemed 'not credible'.

Over the years at university, I was becoming increasingly sick and very fatigued with recurrent bouts of tonsillitis, laryngitis, pharyngitis, with an ulcerated throat, tongue and roof of mouth, and like my heavy periods, they were now every three weeks, (seventeen to twenty-one days), like clockwork. I was constantly in pain, not just in my throat and lower abdomen, but in all my joints, and I felt flu-like symptoms and sickly all the time.

I was unable to breathe properly through my nose, and I frequently took in sharp inhalations through my mouth, like gasping for air. When the Digby Disco once introduced a 'Bubble Machine' to enhance the fun, I was the only one outside choking and desperately trying to breathe.

One morning in a drama class, as I was playing a victim being tied up with a rope, I joked that if I was ever gagged over my mouth with tape in an actual crime scene, I would die before I was rescued!

My throat was so inflamed and constricted, that my glands were the size of golf balls. I was frequently coughing up blood and mucus, and my lungs hurt to inhale. My head and skin burned to the touch, and I was unusually cold. My complexion was always deathly white.

With these symptoms, it is possible that I had died a long time ago…but hadn't realised it. I continued choking in my sleep (sleep apnoea) which disturbed my nights, and I had multiple ear, nose and throat (ENT) infections and I was rarely away from the doctor's surgery.

My GP arranged for me to go on the Contraceptive pill and take Methanoic acid to reduce the period pain, and better enable me to pursue my career in dance.

My GP also left regular prescriptions of antibiotics on the front desk, like clockwork, with the receptionist for me to collect, the bouts so frequent, that I was told by the GP that I didn't need to see him anymore, just "Keep taking the tablets."

I received regular antibiotics, and the doctor advised me every three weeks to also take round the clock paracetamol, and ibuprofen, for the pain.

In January 1996, aged 20 years, I got tonsillitis so badly, that I had a fever of 104*, and the GP prescribed Erythromycin.

I was in my third and final year of university, and my tonsillitis bouts had worsened to the point that my doctor sent me to a hospital ENT 'specialist', who informed me that my tonsils were so badly inflamed that they had actually turned black.

The specialist said that he had never in all his years as a medical practitioner, seen anything like this before and he referred me to have a tonsillectomy (an operation to remove my tonsils). I was put onto a waiting list.

With further research over time, I decided not to have this operation, as there was the potential risk of this directly affecting my singing voice. Plus, the specialist said that because my tonsils were black, they were likely no longer doing their job of protecting my throat. I was now completely intolerant to alcohol. I wanted to join in with all my friends drinking and partying and staying up late, but every time I had even the smallest amount of alcohol, such as a glass of wine, I would be violently sick the following morning, in the strategically placed sink in my student cottage bedroom.

These bouts of vomiting were also now like clockwork, at 8am I would be sick, and by 9am I would be in the splits in the dance studio, with all the other energetic trainee contemporary dancers. I was now used to the sickness and pain - it had become a normal part of living. I was very happy, but very sick, and this combination was frustrating, because being sick all the time, makes you feel utterly drained.

In my final year at university, I was a wreck. I was unable to eat or swallow foods as my throat was so inflamed and my IBS symptoms increasingly more severe, with chronic stomach pains and gastric reflux when I did eat anything.

I was so stressed, that I didn't have time to eat, drink, sleep or rest, and I was not in the least bit hungry. I was producing copious amounts of adrenaline, and it transpires that this was keeping me alert. I was 'tired and wired' with racing thoughts and unable to sleep.

I wasn't hungry at all, and each time I ate food, I became increasingly fatigued post mealtimes, so in order to stay awake and get the high grades I so desperately wanted to achieve, I needed to stay awake!

Friends started to notice my weight loss and my high-speed thoughts and actions, and warned me to take a break and rest, but I didn't have time.

With a type 'A' personality, I was one of the first students to start my dissertation early, researching the subject long before the work had even been set.

I was getting a maximum of one to two hours sleep per night, as my 8,500 - word dissertation deadline loomed and in my perfectionism, I ended up writing over 20,000 words!

My cognitive function was slowing down to an almost zombie-like state, which was ironic because I was so emaciated and white that I looked like one of the 'Walking Dead'.

Every night, I was wide awake in bed, frantically writing up my day's research on my chosen dissertation title, 'Miss Saigon. Can Musical Theatre be considered as High Art?' This was alongside completing two physically and theoretically challenging subjects performing dance and drama by day, and writing everything up by night.

I was unaware of how bad I looked to others, so when my kind-hearted dissertation drama teacher, Viv Riley called me into her office for a meeting to discuss my work, instead of telling me to do more, as she had encouraged others to do, she instructed me to, "Stop everything and watch 'Neighbours'." I couldn't believe my homework, 'Neighbours' lasted twenty-five minutes, and I didn't have twenty-five minutes to spare!

I had no time to sleep, and I couldn't sleep even if I wanted to, as my mind was racing non-stop. I was physically and mentally burnt out, but I knew that "the show must go on!"

On 31st May 1996, I was sitting up in bed choreographing a solo contemporary dance routine, using Laban notation (dance notation) for an upcoming exam, whilst simultaneously learning my script as 'Miss Money Penny' for a comical 'James Bond' musical theatre performance exam the following day. My brain was 'wired' and yet my body was absolutely beyond exhausted.

Sitting upright with pen and paper in hand, I drifted into a semi-conscious state and was roused from this state at 4am, when I suddenly started vomiting.

I moved myself from my slumber to the bedroom sink as fast as I could, and clutching onto the white porcelain frame, I vomited again and again. I consequently became increasingly worried, as I couldn't physically stop being sick. Looking like 'Samara Morgan' from 'The Ring', I dragged my weary waif-like body next door and knocked on my friend and housemate, Lucy Marriott's bedroom door.

I was embarrassed and very apologetic for waking her at this hour. I explained my situation and she immediately jumped out of bed and came to my aid, probably afraid that this apparition before her was going to kill her and put her down a well!

We went back into my bedroom seemingly, to figure out what to do, when I passed out. I was out cold, and to this day I thank my housemates Lucy, Amanda and Paloma, for rescuing me from what could have had a very different outcome. My friends took me to Queen Mary's Hospital, which was fortunately directly across the road from our campus cottage.

I lay in a bed, drifting in and out of consciousness, and when I slowly roused, I felt dazed and confused at my surroundings which were filled with bright lights and a stark white background.

I was now dressed in a white surgical gown. I continued to vomit, baffling the medics surrounding my bed, as to the cause of this illness.

My worried housemates surrounded the bed looking on in horror at their friend's re-enactment of 'The Exorcist!'

I heard a medic ask, "Is she taking any drugs?"

I tried to answer "Yes!" but my housemates laughed and said, "No. Cathy does not take drugs!"

I answered again, 'Yes…tonsillitis drugs!' as I vomited again into another cardboard bowl, hurriedly being placed under my chin by the bedside nurse.

I heard another medic say, "She's gone through fifteen bowls, and she's had two injections in her leg to stop her being sick, but she's still being sick! I don't know why?"

I held onto my agonisingly painful stomach and passed out again, unconscious. This time, I awoke in a lonely dark cupboard of a room all alone, freezing cold and afraid. I had a cannula drip attached to my right arm, and as I roused, I started vomiting again, this time all over myself.

'Help!' I cried, as a nurse came to my aid, carrying more cardboard containers.

'You're in hospital. You have been vomiting for over fifteen hours. We are going to take you for a scan on your stomach today.'

I was beyond exhausted.

"I have to go! I have an exam today…I'm Miss Money Penny," I hurled. The nurse likely thought I was now delusional.

At that moment, my friend and housemate Paloma Forde arrived…

My memory of Cathy being ill was one bizarre night at university, my housemate, Lucy woke me up. We knew that Cathy was not well because she was vomiting and it was really quite bad. She wasn't eating or drinking much. It got worse and worse and the decision was to take her up to hospital.

So, we went up to Queen Mary's hospital, took her in, and we stayed with her for a bit. I remember Cathy having this little dish and being sick and I can remember the colour of it - it was like a yellow green kind of colour. It was definitely unusual; it was like a 'lime green'. Cathy was really poorly and really sick.

We had to go off home, and then in the morning we came to visit her and we came straight up to the hospital to come and see her. I saw a door and it had a star on it and I made Cathy laugh because I came into her room and said, "This door obviously had to be for you, because you are a star!"

Cathy was still really poorly, and I just remember that they couldn't work out what it was. Eventually Cathy got discharged that day, and I do recall that they couldn't work out why she was so poorly.

Cathy was great to live with. She was very energetic, and full of life and a real heart and soul of the party. A huge personality, wonderful humour, a very caring person, wonderful friend. But mainly I remember the energy, she had so much of it!

We just used to have so much fun. She was a very great and loyal friend. She loved to dance and laugh and we always had an amazing time with our singing and dancing - they were probably the best years of my life, my university years, and Cathy was a big part of that!

I do remember if I think of illnesses, of all the people in my years of experience, Cathy is up there as somebody who I have seen, who is really poorly, and it was a different kind of sickness. I just remember that because of the colour of the vomit. It definitely wasn't right.

Paloma Forde – Founder of Screening4dyslexia, Teacher and University flatmate

CHAPTER TWELVE: Startle ME
Terrifyingly Entertaining!

"Times of stress are also times that are signals for growth, and if we use adversity properly, we can grow through adversity." - Rabbi Dr Abraham Twerski.

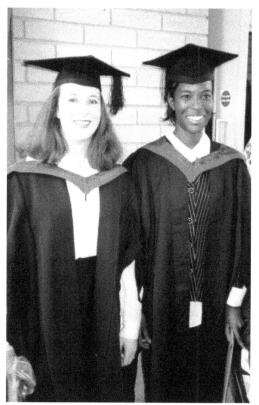

Catherine Vandome at 'The University Of Surrey' Graduation Ceremony with dancer Susanne Marston, on the 25th July, 1996.

On Wednesday 18th January 1995, Cathy and I went to Alien War Zone at the Trocadero in Piccadilly Circus.
Alien War Zone is a re-creation of the Alien films where a group of guides escort you through various scenes from the Alien Film. Cathy and I stupidly thought this would be a good way to spend our afternoon. "It will be a laugh," we said.
There were about ten of us in our group, including a little boy who was shaking from fear from the very start. As we were waiting for our turn to go in, a lady burst out of the venue at full pelt, grabbed hold of a pillar for support and slumped to the ground in a heap. She looked like she had been chased by a pack of wild dogs!

It was our turn to go in and we were guided past alien eggs that were awaiting to hatch, and led into a room where we were told to, "Sit down and shut up!" The guide left us alone to go on ahead and check if it was safe. Up until this point we had not been scared, but something about being left in a dark room with a door at each end, where you knew an alien could burst through at any point, became terrifying.

All of a sudden, the guide burst into the room and told us to get out quickly. At the same time through the other door, burst a massive alien. Everyone jumped up and started to run. I was so scared (even though I knew the alien was just a man in a suit). I couldn't even move from fear, and when I did manage to get up, everyone was trying to run through the door at the same time. I was running so fast I couldn't stop, and ran straight into a wall. I hurt my knee so badly, I could barely walk. There were tears in my eyes and all I wanted to do was go home.

Outside the room, everyone was running so fast away from the alien. I saw Cathy fall over and about five fifteen-year-old boys just trampled straight over her back. One person crushed her hand under foot. Her front teeth hit the floor. I saw a massive alien standing over her. I kept thinking about what I would tell her mum! "Sorry Cathy won't be coming home, she got carried off by a seven-foot alien!"

Somehow, I made it out of there on my own, without Cathy. The alien carried her off. All of us collapsed outside, just like the lady we had seen when we were waiting to go in.

Then we saw the security guards watching the whole saga on the security T.V. and they were absolutely wetting themselves laughing at us. Cathy finally emerged out of a side door and we both limped off to Queen Mary's Hospital A&E to get our injuries treated. The doctors found it hilarious when we explained we had been injured trying to run away from a seven-foot alien. Alien War Zone eventually got closed down due to so many people getting hurt.

Love you!

Susanne Marston - Cathy's friend from Roehampton University, University of Surrey - Administrator and Fitness Instructor

Terrified, I race with the group away from the seven-foot heavy breathing grey and black alien, dripping fluid from its teeth.

Running fast inside, Alien War Zone, I suddenly lose my balance, and fall face down onto the criss-crossed steel metal gridded floor with a thud, chipping my front tooth. Screaming to safety, members of the group run over the top of my body, where I am left positioned in a theatrical, murder-mystery dead-body pose with arms and legs extended.

Alone and frozen in fear, I blink and very slowly open my eyes. I am inside an eerie, cold, dark room with smoke machines billowing, my body battered and bruised from the mass of footprints across my back, and I notice a stiletto indentation in the centre of my bleeding left hand. I can feel the presence of something looming over me and breathing heavily, and I cautiously turn my bleeding head to look over my left shoulder. The Seven-Foot Alien is staring down at me! Sheer terror grips me, and like Little Red Riding Hood, I stutter "Ppplease, don't eat me!"

Well, that must have made the actors day! The man dressed as an Alien vanished, and allowed me to hobble out and try to find the rest of my group. The hospital doctor examined my wounds in the cubicle adjacent to my friend, Susanne, and he laughingly asked, "Did you not know the Alien wasn't real?"

Still shaking and traumatised, I replied, "Doctor, that Alien was real!"

The doctor and I both laughed.

My friend, Susanne and I link arms in sympathy, leaving the hospital, and hobble away for ice cream. We both vow never to tell anyone about this experience for fear of being laughed at...until now!

A few months later, Susanne and I were ready for our next entertainment challenge. This time on Streatham Ice rink. After an initial cautionary skate around the smooth, circular, cold, sheer ice rink, we were both in our element.

The rink was relatively quiet, which gave us more space.

We found our ballet training enabled our ability to balance on the ice, and through lots of laughter we were enjoying a fun afternoon perfecting basic skating tricks.

Susanne stopped at the side of the rink for a brief rest.

"See you in a minute!" I hollered, speeding off at top speed, laughing at the exhilaration from the adrenaline rush. I raced around the rink, and I was back with Susanne in moments, after completing my first lap, and as I zoomed past her she giggled at my speed. Unbeknownst to me, a group of teenage boys had entered the ice and were hanging around the side of the rink, near Susanne. I was on my second lap, ever increasing in speed, when suddenly my ice skate hit something hard on the ground and I flipped high in the air, and landed hard on the ice with a 'crack'. I lay flat on my back on the ice, momentarily dazed and shocked as to what had just happened.

Susanne instantly rushed to my aid. As I stood up, searing in pain, I heard laughter coming from nearby, where the boys were standing.

"Come with me, Cathy," Susanne said, whilst gently helping me to my feet, and off the rink to safety.

Once outside, Susanne explained that she saw one of the boys purposefully extend his leg to trip me up on the ice. Our entertaining afternoon of 'Dancing on Ice' became 'Dancing in Ice' and we once more found comfort at the local ice cream parlour.

My ex-boyfriend set regular challenges in our relationship. Our dates were very much like 'Squid Games.'

"Cathy, I dare you to jump off the very top of the swimming pool diving board," he challenged me.

"Ok!" I laughed, thinking that this had to be quite an easy feat.

I had recently managed to fly my hundred-pound birthday gift from him, a remote-controlled aeroplane, from the top of Greenwich Park hill, into the abyss, defying gravity whilst obeying the laws of aerodynamics. This was the most expensive few seconds of laughter, that I have ever had. I had also successfully achieved his previous week's challenge, skiing from the very top of a London dry ski slope, all the way to the bottom without falling, on a first attempt.

I was grateful for my one dry ski slope lesson, at Pontins in childhood.

I say lesson - my dad, two brothers and I, were standing in a vertical line in large skies, when my dad accidentally fell sideways knocking us all over like a 'Vandome domino rally'. This was to my mother's amusement, as she was safely taking photographs at the bottom of the slope, not positioned as I was, at the bottom of the domino rally.

Afraid of heights, but always up for a new challenge, I climbed higher and higher up the vertical ladders with a racing heart, feeding off the adrenaline.

Once at the top, I looked down at the Lego-sized swimming pool and people below, and my heart made a stark warning 'thud' sound. Standing at the edge of the highest pale blue wobbling diving board, wearing a pink bikini, the male pool attendant looked up and gestured for me to 'jump'.

My body froze, as my gut bellowed, "No!"

"I can't do it!" my teeth chattered, as I stepped aside, and let the athletic man behind me leap like a gazelle off the top with ease.

"Come on Cathy! I'm going to jump off too, its easy!" my ex-boyfriend shouted up to me encouragingly, from the safety of two ladders down. I walked back to the front of the diving board and gulped. I hated failing anything. I had to do this challenge. I was becoming increasingly more afraid the longer I stood in anticipation. By now, the laughing pool attendant had cajoled a number of spectators below to shout up to me to "Go for it!" People were whistling, and slow hand clapping, believing that I was dumb enough to jump off.

"It's now or never!" my ex-boyfriend shouted up.

With that I jumped. I don't know how, as I was terrified of heights, but I jumped. I didn't dive, as I should have done, I jumped feet first, and as the soles of my feet hit the water, it felt like I was jumping through an iced block.

"Ouch!" I screamed silently, as every bone felt broken travelling through the ice-cold water, and I sank deeper and deeper and deeper.

I had held my breath as I landed, but my lungs hurt, and I suddenly felt as though I didn't have enough oxygen to get back up to the surface.

"I am going to drown," I thought.

I pushed with every bit of the weakened body strength I could muster to resurface. The other people made diving look easy. I didn't have the strength to get back up. As I floated slowly upwards, frantically waving my arms, I recalled my childhood where I had almost drowned aged nine, in the wave machine at The Sandcastle in Blackpool, dragged out by my right arm, up and out of the pool, by the astute poolside attendant.

My mind then raced to my late teens in an outdoor hotel pool in Greece, where after winning the evening's competition of, 'Who can run across the most lilos in the swimming pool in a row', and managing a surprising twelve, I next swam under a lilo awaiting the next race. This lilo was then jumped on by an unknowing couple, and I was left circling like 'Jaws' underneath, but without the gills to breathe. The holiday rep spotted me and pulled me out of the water into the resuscitation position. Today was going to be my hat trick.

I resurfaced literally just in time, and promptly nearly passed out. The pool side attendant came to my aid, his laughter had now turned to grave concern. I was helped out of the pool, where my body was shaking, and teeth chattering, as I desperately tried to fill my constricted lungs with air. I looked deathly white naturally, so spectators would be forgiven for thinking that I was actually dead!

My skin complexion was so white, that my dear and hilarious friend, Rolph Patterson, once correctly observed that when I sunbathe with my eyes closed…I look like I have been embalmed!

I looked up and saw my ex-boyfriend clambering back down the ladders to safety. After watching me, he decided that this challenge was quite literally 'death defying entertainment'.

Years later, I was watching the Spanish Hotel Cabaret Entertainers, when I noticed my next terrifying challenge I wished to overcome.

"Stand very still and hold the pythons head away from your face," the hotel photographer instructed me, as he wrapped a huge, weighty python around my small neck and shoulders. The python could hear that my heartbeat was twice as fast as the other guests, and he looked as uneasy as I felt.

"Smile," said the photographer.

"Smile?" I thought. "Is he talking to me, or the snake?"

For his amusement, the photographer stood back and let the python wrap its large dry scaly body around mine, as I squealed and froze in fear. The packed family audience now started watching me instead of the hotel entertainment. My sheer fear generated abounding laughter from the hotel guests, and of course it gave the photographer the focus he needed to generate more customers. I once played 'Kaa, the Snake,' but I never thought that one day I would be wearing him!

In the same way, years later, when NLP Co-founder, Dr Richard Bandler, challenged me, within his NLP course, to hold a large black tarantula in my hand, I embraced the challenge with the same amount of fear, but this time in so doing, I genuinely overcame my lifelong fear of spiders.

After years of a poor diet, multiple highly athletic challenges, and after successfully handling reptiles, I was now equipped for the 'I'm a Celebrity Jungle'.

"Thank you for this birthday treat to Alton Towers, Leanne!" I squeal, as we climb into the first big rollercoaster ride, side by side, and pull down the safety bar above.

"You're welcome!" My talented dancer friend, Leanne Kirkham shouts, above the loud thumping music. "I absolutely love rides!"

"I don't, I'm terrified!" I laugh.

"Then why did you choose Alton Towers?" Leanne asks laughing.

"I love being terrified!" I giggle.

We go on every single ride, racing up and down, back and forth, round and round, and about half way around the theme park, as we are hanging vertically from the bar, about to drop, Leanne laughingly asks "Cathy, are there any rides today, where you have actually opened your eyes?"

"No! But this is the best birthday gift ever!" I gasp, with eyes tightly shut!

We both belly laugh at the absurdity of choosing to spend your birthday absolutely terrified and in the dark! I hadn't realised that I was actually addicted to adrenaline, and like sugar, I craved more.

Sometime later, I was booked to work as an actress for the Lancashire Constabulary for a number of Police training days, in my hometown of Fulwood, in Preston. I arrived at the local Police Station cast as a 'Group Four Officer', suited in a white blouse and black pencil skirt, with my hair tied up in a bun.

I hadn't been fully briefed on my acting days ahead, and although I was advised to bring any theatrical stage make up for the application of blood and bruises, I simply naively followed instructions.

Once inside the police station, I laughed along with my fellow actors about the absurdity of the acting job, working with two genuine police officers playing criminals. A second female actress, proceeded to read the script brief to me, whilst I applied our make-up wounds. The basic subtext was that both of the Police officers were playing escaped convicted prisoners, who had captured both myself and the other actress, (playing the police van driver), as we took the two prisoners to another prison site. We were directed throughout by the Lancashire Police, from within the station by telephone, and we were told to remain quiet at intermittent intervals, as the outside police officers enacted a training day raid of the building. We were instructed to open the front door and begin live improvisation on cue, and re-enact the unfolding drama.

I was in my element, laughing away and enjoying the set up and telephone demands over the indoor telephone to the outside awaiting police officers, unaware of the drama unfolding outdoors.

I had totally underestimated the intensity of the situation, and it hit me hard as the front door was flung open and the large, acting police officer, now clad in a black balaclava, grabbed my tiny waist and put a real black hand gun to my head, shouting, "I will shoot to kill her if you don't all back away from the building!"

As I looked outside of the front door, I was surrounded by a sea of large, uniformed, armed Police Officers all pointing guns in my direction and shouting, 'Drop your weapon, or we will fire!'

I was absolutely terrified. My blood ran cold and I acted afraid, screaming, 'Help me!"

The scene played out, and the front door was repeatedly opened and closed as the improvisation unfolded, with more stage make up of liquid blood and bruises being applied to my face, between scenes. Eventually, I was directed to leave the building from a side door, with the criminal holding me tightly by his large, thick-set arms around my neck, before throwing me onto the floor.

I was thrown down by the excitable acting Police Officer, whom had taken his part very seriously indeed. With a gun pointed at the back of my head by him, and numerous guns pointing my way from the oncoming sea of blue and black costumes, I didn't need to act terrified.

I continued to crawl away on my knees, whilst holding my shaking hands above my head, as per the awaiting police officer's instructions. I momentarily stopped breathing, keeping in character until the armed police officers rescuing me, eventually came to my aid.

It took several minutes before I heard a police officer say, "You can stop acting now love! Bloody hell, you were the best actor we have ever seen! You looked genuinely terrified! Well done, you deserve your days fee! Honestly you looked terrified!"

I slowly lifted my head, breathless, with tears uncontrollably rolling down both cheeks, and said, "I'm not acting. I am terrified!"

"Get her a cup of tea! Quickly!" I heard the Police officer instruct another.

"I can't do this again tomorrow, I'm sorry. My heart is racing. I'm too frightened, I'm so sorry."

"Yes, you can love, you're the best actress we've ever had, and we will redirect it so that you leave the building a different way, if you're afraid of looking at a large group of armed police officers!"

The following day, as per the director's instructions, once the front door flung open, I closed my eyes and I pretended to pass out on the ground. This time I was stretchered off by two police officers, so that I didn't have to look at anyone in this terrifying armed combat police scene!

For longevity of life, I decided it was a bright idea to never audition for a horror film, from now on I had best stick to comedy!

On 25th July 1996, I graduated from The University of Surrey with a 2/1 BA (Hons) Degree in Dance and Drama.

Despite the headed warnings from my contemporary dance teacher; "Cathy! Stop looking at the audience when you dance. You're not dancing on a cruise ship!" I was inspired by her to follow my own dreams.

Three days after my graduation ceremony, I proudly took to the seas and began dancing on a cruise ship, performing in Musical Theatre productions on board Sun Cruise's, MS. Seawing.

Dancer, actor, now author! What next for Miss Vanderflange?
Where to start with the bundle of energy and laughter that is Cathy? I was fortunate enough to study drama with Cathy at university, and I can't think of a time with her when we weren't laughing.
Cathy really is a one off. She has an unquenchable passion for life and a boundless drive and determination to succeed. She is caring, funny, unpredictable, fearless, charming and utterly lovable.
She was there when I needed a friend and vice versa.
We had so much fun, nightclubbing at Carwash nightclub in London, turning, "Can you feel the force?" song lyrics into, "Can you feel the horse?" with accompanying dance moves; causing chaos at 'The Clothes Show' and ending up

at 'The Marriott hotel' afterwards joking with the band that played there, and being surrounded by 90s fashion favourites.

Quietly meditating during yoga and her surprising me with a boob grab and us muffling uncontrollable giggles until the end of the session, Cathy was the Marion to my Danton in our university theatre production, 'Danton's Death' by Georg Buchner. I have so many memories, all of them fond, and all with a northern chuckle in the background.

I can remember one time when Cathy wasn't well and she ended up in hospital. Even then I remember her still cracking jokes and never wanting to be any trouble. Now when her life and all the success that she built has been utterly turned on its head, it's no surprise that Cathy is putting that drive into helping others and getting well. She's unstoppable!

Cathy has a lust for life that is rare to find, and the talent to tackle it. I admire her wholeheartedly for everything that she has achieved and have no doubt she will continue to achieve. I can't wait to find out what she does next!

Good luck Miss Vanderflange! Lots of love always, Jane xxx

Jane Shelley - Actress

CHAPTER THIRTEEN: All aboard with ME
All at Sea!

"You ME and the sea." - Elizabeth Haynes.

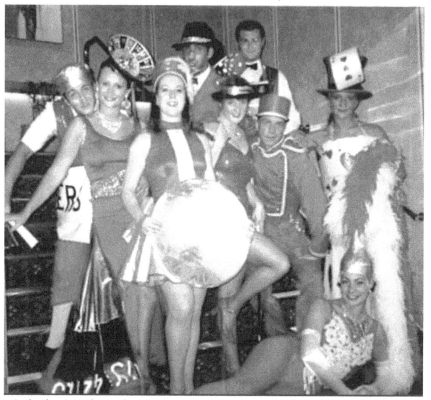

Catherine Vandome dancing on board Suncruises 'MS Seawing' Cruiseship, with Dance Captain Jo Boase, Rachel Green - Ainslie, Joseph Koniak, Victoria Potter, Robert Maskell, Hannah Simmonds, Jeff Sturgess, Susie Schaeffer and Newley Aucutt for Adam Wide's 'Openwide Productions', 1996.

Cathy joined our existing team on the MS Seawing in 1996, and her energy and enthusiasm hit us like a bouncy ball. She loved to dance, actually she loved doing anything that was required in her daily roles as cruise staff/entertainer.

Cathy conducted a bridge tour like a historian would recount a famous battle, keeping the guests' attention, which was not an easy task!

Cathy thrived in this environment and was such a pleasure to be around, her happiness rubbed off on us all.

What we didn't realise was what a strong and resilient person she was, she is a true inspiration for us all. Love you Cathy x

Rachel Green-Ainslie - Cruise Director and Entertainer

The deafening sound of the huge engine fired up, and within minutes we were gliding slowly upwards through the misty clouds and into the piercing, clear blue skies above.

Filled with anticipation and excitement, I thanked the musical production choreographer, Steven Baker, seated beside me, for giving me the opportunity to perform on board the MS Seawing. As we glided through the air, Steven told me that the onboard Entertainment Team had to be able to dance, sing, act, compare, have all round versatility, a fun personality, and great PR skills, to be able to work with others. I laughed and asked, "Then why am I sitting here?"

Steven told me that out of more than a hundred hopefuls auditioning, one of the reasons that they had chosen me for the position, was because I had made the panel laugh. He explained that when Adam Wide from 'Openwide Productions', had recalled me and invited me to script read in front of the audition panel, performing 'Maybelline' from their production of 'Route 66', that he was demonstrating how the character was to be played in an American accent, when I had replied, "I thought you said it was American?"

"That was the exact moment we chose you," he laughed.

I was very flattered indeed to be considered funny. This was the definitive professional compliment, which helped sow the seed of my eventually becoming a stand-up comedian. We landed in Palma Majorca, and I was taken over the rickety gang plank to meet the Entertainment Team, on board the large bright white and blue cruise ship.

'What a truly magical experience', I thought, 'I am fulfilling my dream.'

As I took in the surrounding: the sunshine, the ship, and the sea, I smiled broadly, as I generously applied my factor fifty suncream. Here I was, aged twenty-one, about to travel around the world, whilst doing the job I loved! I was replacing a lead dancer at very short notice, and I had only three days and nights, to learn every single production number, before my opening night. Every evening was jam packed full of entertainment, there was dancing, singing and acting in the Musical Theatre productions, including a show called 'Picture House' and another called 'Route 66.'

There were also cabaret spots with comparing and singing, plus nightly musical song and dance routines, to open the shows for the guest stand-up comedians, magicians and other specialist acts on board. I watched the guest acts religiously, particularly the stand ups' ease and confidence with which they performed, from their microphone technique, to the delivery of the jokes they told, and how they moved on stage and spoke directly to the audience.

I wished that I had their confidence to stand up on stage alone, and talk into a microphone. One of our musical productions had thirteen costume changes per show, with two shows in one night. That's twenty-six costume changes. I spent more time backstage taking my clothes on and off!

How my brain absorbed so many fast complex dance routines and musical production numbers, in such a short period of time, I will never know - I was practising all day and night to perfect them. We worked all day doing on board leisure activities with the guests, and all afternoon and evening on stage, and I routinely capped around three to five hours sleep per night. I would get into bed at 3am, after post-performance dancing for pleasure in the Crow's Nest disco, and be up at 8am for 'Good Morning-Sea Stretch', running a morning aerobics class for the sober, elderly passengers on board.

'Life is a Cabaret! I will sleep when I'm old,' I thought.

I was honoured to be working with incredibly multi-talented entertainers, including my dance partner Joseph Koniak, Anthony Bristoe, Louise Byron, Rachel Green-Ainslie, Michelle Anderton, Jo Boase, Victoria Potter, Jeff Sturgess, Robert Maskell, Joff Eaton, Morgan Van Selman, and many others, who taught me so much about the art of stage craft, and I was blessed that we all became life-long friends.

The choreography was very slick and professional, and the talented Dance Captain, Jo Boase was incredible, working hard to teach me so many routines, in such a short period of time. I felt so happy. My nervous system was cranked up to the max. Adrenaline pumping and excitement bursting, with a euphoric high that no drug could ever match! I was so excited to be sailing across the Mediterranean Sea, preparing to open the musical medley production with five other girls dressed in black sequinned 1920's style dresses, performing 'Dancing Fool' from the hit musical 'Copacabana'.

Life cannot get any better than this!

I had recently prepared for my travels, by having my B.C.G. vaccination booster, which having previously failed this with an allergic reaction at high school, I was now told by my GP that it was compulsory for travel. I was given a test dose on 18th July 1996, and the full dose on 25th July just prior to flying.

Fourteen days later, on 3rd August, I was celebrating my 22nd birthday with fellow entertainers, after our evening musical performances, when I suddenly couldn't breathe. I started having a severe anaphylactic choking episode. I genuinely thought that was it, as I fell to the floor holding my throat, gasping for air, by the Clipper lounge show bar. I had encountered a number of these choking episodes throughout my life, but this one I distinctly remember, because I thought that I was going to die on my birthday, halfway around the Mediterranean Sea, and I hadn't yet had time to disembark and see the sights!

After I regained my full faculties, and I could breathe again, fellow entertainers proceeded to make me laugh, saying that, 'If anyone dies on board, they are put into the fridge freezer, and we all get extra ice cream. So, if we all get served ice cream tomorrow, we know what's happened to Cathy!"

I read the mornings itinerary, 'CATHY: 8.30AM - SEA STRETCH AEROBICS, 9AM, 10AM, 11AM, 2PM - BRIDGE TOURS'

I laughed, "OK, is this a joke? I'm doing a whole day of Bridge Tours!"

"Well, you shouldn't be so good at them," my Entertainment Team Leader, Morgan Van Selman replied, with a cheeky smile. By day, the Entertainment Team turned into an onboard cast of 'Hi-de-Hi'.

I wore a crisp white shirt and ruffled white knee length skirt, with royal blue court shoes, and a royal blue blazer, with cruise ship epaulettes on my shoulders. Our daytime duties included playing deck quoits, shuffleboard, darts and carpet bowls with the passengers, and the games became even more adventurous when the ship swayed. There was 'Sunday by the Sea', where we dressed in brightly coloured 1920's swimsuits and matching hats, with the compare egging on the sunbathing passengers to have us all pushed into the upper deck swimming pool. We also had a fun filled audience participation 'Country and Western' themed event, with dancing, singing and comedy.

I found that whenever I was playing the saucy barmaid, 'Lilo Lil', the wives would stop their husbands from country dancing with me, so I much preferred playing the little old dancing 'Grandma', once more letting my GCSE drama teacher know that you *can* make a professional career out of playing old ladies!

I hosted a weekly deck quiz, which was a great opportunity to develop my comparing and microphone skills, later used on stage as a solo singer. One of the quiz book questions I read aloud, was "Can you dislocate your jaw kissing?" The surrounding elderly ladies giggled, and laughed even louder when I revealed that the quiz answer was, "Yes, and that this had genuinely happened to me!"

> *"I had the pleasure of working with Cathy on the cruise ships. I will always remember her bubbly personality, good humour and sense of fun.*
>
> *My fondest memory of her is when she sang. I always admired her charming, comedic banter in between songs.*
>
> *Spending so much time together at sea certainly helped us forged lasting friendships, but once you have met Cathy, you will never forget her! She has a buzzing energy that is very contagious!!*
>
> *Making a living in the entertainment industry is hard enough, but having to do so with a health condition too, must be debilitating. Cathy's strength of character is a force to be reckoned with and she is truly an inspiration to others."*
>
> **Michelle Anderton - Singer/Dancer**

On Sunday mornings we religiously visited our 'Muster Stations' armed with bright orange life jackets, and we would demonstrate to our designated passenger group how to put these on in an emergency. One nervous middle-aged lady asked me, "Cathy, will you travel all the way down to this lower deck to save us in an emergency?"

"Not a chance! It's every man for himself, I shall be jumping overboard!"

The lady belly-laughed at this, and had no idea that I was serious.

All the day time activities were fun and games - all except 'Bridge Tours'. Nobody wanted to do Bridge Tours.

To make the Bridge Tours more interesting, I learned as much of the entire layout of the cruise ship Bridge as possible, and subconsciously turned it into a comedy routine. I studied the inner workings of the Bridge in great detail, with the complicated multi-coloured dashboard of numerous controls and levers, and I explained to the enthusiastic passengers what each one did, warning, "Whatever you do, don't touch the red button!"

I smiled, as one by one they shifted nervously away from the 'red button', not asking what it did or even realising that I was joking! I explained that the cruise ship has three engines, and I pointed to starboard, stern, port and bow, which became useful information to learn and use in later years, as a children's drama game set onboard a cruise ship!

With the Bridge empty and running on cruise control, and the Captain sitting outside, I would joke to the passengers that, "The Captain was outside sleeping, and that no one was steering the ship." Despite being in the middle of the Mediterranean ocean, I always ended the tour with an adrenaline boosting cry of, "Iceberg ahead!" The reactions were priceless!

"I'm so sorry I can't do a forward roll."

"Everyone can do a forward roll," the Dance Captain laughed.

As a perfectionist, I tried my best, and Jo quickly realised that although I could do a double pirouette in high heels, I couldn't do a basic forward roll, for it somehow hurt my neck and knocked me dizzy with vertigo.

"Right,' she said supportively, "You're at the front of the dance routine for 'Five Guys Named MO' and when we all land on each other's back, I'm going to help you by pushing you into the forward roll! Oh! and you're wearing a trilby!"

We both laughed.

The opening night of this energetic and highly physical dance routine, ended with my landing on the corner of the stage with a 'clunk', as the bottom of my jaw hit the metal framed stage edge.

As the blood trickled down my chin, I carried on smiling and leapt off the front of the stage with the other dancers, into the finale freeze frame position. I was later given sutures under my chin, and advised to rest, but that word was not in my vocabulary. My underlying balance issues were now heightened by the motion of the ocean, but at least now I could pass them off as normal.

The following week in my tap-dancing routine, I rolled over so badly on my ankle that it swelled black and blue. Surprisingly it didn't break, but I couldn't get my dance shoes on. Getting my dance shoes on was far more important than the pain, for "The show must go on."

Behind the twenty-four-hour entertainment smile, I was regularly unwell and increasingly tired, but I would push myself harder to try to keep up with the stamina of everyone else. There were the odd occasions when I quite literally could not get out of bed, and times when I strangely couldn't physically move. The entertainment team leader, Morgan, popped his head in to check on me inside my cabin bed, and he announced how many bridge tours I was missing that day, and how disappointed the passengers would be, to try to cheer me up! He knew that I wasn't a shirker, and I saw genuine concern on his face for my wellbeing. I rarely drank any alcohol, as it made me so sick, and I was perhaps getting my euphoric high from yet another round of tonsillitis medication.

We always knew in advance if the seas were going to be exceptionally rocky, as sick bags lined the golden side rails of the Clipper Lounge, where the onboard theatre was. Despite the turbulent weather conditions, the productions still went on, unless it was so bad that pieces of the set flew across the stage. One night, half a car from the production of 'Route 66' rolled across the stage into the wings, and the curtain came down.

'Thud'

My television crash lands on my bright blue carpeted cabin floor.

"Ouch!"

I tip sideways out of the top bed bunk and join it.

Knock Knock!

My cabin door flings open, as I see various cabin crew frantically running around.

"We are letting everyone know that this is an emergency and tonight's show is cancelled. The ship's engine has stopped, and we are bobbing about in the middle of the Mediterranean Sea."

The ship is tipping vigorously forwards and backwards, forwards and backwards, sending everyone and everything within it flying.

I learn that the restaurant and bars had crashed, and that some of the crew were doing wheelies across the floor. I also learned that any passengers who had been injured, were now being airlifted out from the top of the ship above the Crow's Nest.

Weak at the knees, bobbing back and forth, I hold onto the wooden grip rail and attempt to climb the stairs, which I find to be an enormous physical challenge.

I eventually join my fellow entertainers in the crew mess and watch them laughingly trying to eat their bowls of soup, as they up end on their laps, and their chair tips backwards.

The onboard stand-up comedian tells me not to worry, and that as I'm only little, I can use him as a life raft. This brings a little bit of colour back into my even whiter with fear filled cheeks.

I realise at this moment that in times of extreme fear, my family and I instantaneously go into 'flight mode' rather than 'fight mode'. The Vandome family would be best used as 'human hand grenades' on a battlefield.

I am warned that we may have to exit the cruise ship in the designated life rafts, for with one engine down, if the weather turns into a storm, we will most likely tip over.

The fear of this real life 'Titanic' experience unfolding, has gripped my ability to move my legs, so there is no way that I will be climbing down three flights of stairs to my Muster Station, to collect Mrs Smith and show her how to blow her own whistle!

"Did you say that one engine was down?" I ask.

"Yes."

"Well, there are three engines on a ship, so if one goes down there are still another two to get us back to dry land." My Bridge Tours had not been in vain.

Just then, the Captain announces, "Although the ship is rocking back and forth, the weather is extremely calm, and it won't be long before we are back sailing again."

Once docked at our next destination, I spot deep sea divers swimming down underneath the ship, to save the day.

I travelled all around the Mediterranean Sea and the Atlantic Ocean, with opportunities on my days off, to enjoy the tourist excursions and see the incredible sights. In the Mediterranean, amongst many other sites, I visited St Peter's Cathedral in Rome, The Casino de Monte-Carlo in Monaco, went down The Monte toboggan, (Carros de Cesto) in Madeira, and up La Rambla in Barcelona.

In the Caribbean, after a whole week at sea, absolutely everybody on board wanted to visit all of the islands, with their white sands, steel bands, palm trees and clear blue seas. With all the passengers and most of the staff disembarked, I questioned why on earth one single man wanted to stay onboard and play indoor darts on my daytime activity, when we had just arrived in Barbados? I instinctively knew why he was single. The 'icing on the cake' for me, was when my parents came on board for a Caribbean cruise with a magical team of my fellow entertainers, and I. As seasoned professional cruisers, having been on board some of the biggest cruise ships around the world, my parents enjoyed every minute and said, "Well it might not be the biggest, but it is certainly one of the best!" I secretly hoped they meant me.

> "I first met Cathy somewhere at sea and we hit it off straight away - a northern girl with a huge heart and always full of fun.
> We performed together in various musical productions and often played the same comedy roles! We both rocked the granny costume for 'Country and Western event afternoon!'
> Cathy and I also duetted with the resident pianist in the ship's cocktail lounge.
> On Easter Monday, Cathy introduced me to the 'Egg Rolling'. This tradition was unfamiliar to me, but we did laugh whilst rolling our Easter eggs down the decks of a cruise ship in Barbados!
> Great memories of a fantastic time!"
> **Louise Byron - Dancer/Singer**

Wearing a swimsuit and full black scuba diving equipment, armed with no formal safety training, unless you count putting on the heavily weighted scuba diving gear and falling backwards onto the floor as 'formal' practise, I was the last to tip backwards out of the little anchored bobbing white boat, into the clear blue Caribbean Sea in Grenada.

I begged the young instructor, and I say instructor in the loosest terms, to "Hold my hand underwater, and don't let go," as I had absolutely no idea how to operate any of the equipment, in order to get back up without getting the bends!

My fellow entertainers in the excursion, had some prior understanding of what to do, and fortunately for them, I was now swimming alongside the instructor, inhaling a combination of 78% nitrogen, 21% oxygen, and 1% trace gasses, leading the way, and acting as a beacon of light to the group, as my skin illuminated fluorescent white underwater, enhanced (only slightly) by wearing factor 50 suncream!

A huge manta ray swam overhead. If I had known that was a shark, I would not have kept my eyes open. The instructor took me further and further away from the group, until eventually all that I could see and feel ahead, was dark black icy cold water. He gave me a sign underwater to let go of his hand, likely so that the blood could flow to his fingers, but I squeezed it even tighter, so he had no choice, but to get me back up to safety. After he operated the scuba diving equipment for me, and got me back up to the boat alive, he laughed and told me that we had just travelled forty metres under, on a first dive! This excursion certainly sounded very legal and safe to me!

Luckily, I didn't get the bends, but I knew I must have been round the bend to have participated in a potential 'Jaws' remake as Susan Backlinie's short, white, northern stunt double!

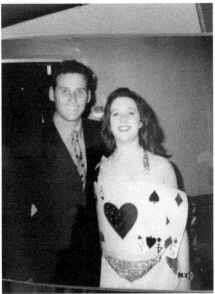

Catherine Vandome as the 'Dolly Dealer' in
'Play your cards right' with Anthony Bristoe,
onboard Suncruises 'MS Seawing' in 1996.

Miss Catherine Van Der May and I met in 1996 sailing the oceans around the Mediterranean, Aegean and Black seas and also around the Americas, as part of the Sun Cruises entertainment team.
I was a singer/actor and came back as a dancer/singer/actor as they really put us through our paces! We were both twenty-one at the time and living our best lives (although at the time we didn't really know it).
We had so much fun and dramas on board the ship of dreams!

From the moment Cathy and I met, we hit it off straight away. I was obviously very funny and charming and could sing, and Cathy was happy that people laughed at her jokes!

Cathy was also a force to be reckoned with - she can sing, dance and is naturally a very funny lady. She's a person anyone can instantly warm to. She has the ability to make a very dull day so sunny, and we had a few on our travels, but Cathy made it all the more bearable when she would break the ice by making fun or light of any situation!

We have continued to remain loyal, lifelong friends and she has always stuck by me in times of trouble and self-doubt. Cathy has always had the ability to lift my spirits when needed…that is Cathy Vandome…a loving, caring, selfless, uber talented passionate human…who also tells jokes!

When we left our cruise life behind, we both had dreams and ambitions of making it to the West End stage…via The London Dungeons on Tooley Street! We went with friends for a day out and ended up booking ourselves jobs after chatting to staff and getting an audition for the 'Gruesome Characters.'

I did a sterling audition as a 'drunk 18th Century Judge'…full wig and hammer. Whilst Cathy was an excellent 'Lady of the night', visiting the Ten Bells Pub and flirting with Jack the Ripper!

We lasted less than twenty-four hours in the job, after seeing a member of staff get punched for scaring his girlfriend. I wasn't sure it was the place for us!

Skip forward a few years when Cathy started getting symptoms. It's very hard to sit and watch your close, energetic, bubbly, spirited friend, struggle to make sense of what the future was holding for her.

How Cathy has learnt to deal and cope with the horrendous situation she has found herself in - feeling trapped, paralysed, wheelchair bound for many years. To lose her life, her dreams and Performing Arts school, which she has taken years to build. It's just unimaginable! But Cathy being Cathy wasn't taking any of this lying down…or sitting in a wheelchair!

The sheer determination and work she has done with Dr Perrin, to bring her diagnosis to the forefront with such humour and grace is amazing, and should be applauded…for she is nothing short of a miracle. I thank her for being in my life and reminding me that we are not going to be beaten down by anything! Love you darling x

Anthony Bristoe - Singer/Performer and Events/Butler. Twenty-five years working in the West End for giants like Sir Cameron Macintosh and Loyd Andrew Lloyd Webber in various roles.

CHAPTER FOURTEEN: Wait on ME

All Actors are waiters waiting to be seen!

"Los Angeles is peopled by waiters and carpenters and drivers who are there to be actors." - Patrick Duffy.

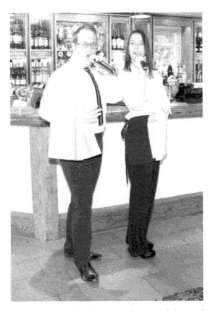

Catherine Vandome as a 'Singing Waiter' with Male Vocalist and Exclusively Elton Tribute - Mark Anthony Tedin, in 2013.

I met Cathy in 2004 at Stage Coach Theatre School in Preston. Cathy was the drama teacher and Leanne Kirkham was the dance teacher - both super cute, funky, young and full of laughs! - the kind of northern British laughs with jokes that took me a while to understand…one needs to catch the accent and inflection to really cotton on, but as an Aussi/born U.K. resident, having worked in Clitheroe for a year, I think I got most of it! The rhetoric was funny, energetic and most memorably - so welcoming to me.

Cathy came into my life that day and we became close colleagues, and then great friends. Cathy came to work with me in my school, which I had established in Clitheroe, 'The Schiller Academy of Performing Arts' that happily and successfully provided a very high-quality tuition to the regional area Clitheroe, and the beautiful Ribble Valley of Lancashire.

Cathy's energy was 'electric' every week, wherever she went - as a performer, teacher, collaborator, advocate and complete artist. She never missed a beat. We communicated consistently for all our planning, developing the student's talents, and enhancing their performance techniques and interests.

Cathy's laugh and comedic slant on practically everything was infectious, always such an absolutely refreshing joy to be around.

Cathy became a true friend and a person I could trust 100%. Cathy was also 100% reliable, compassionate, kind, sincere and also wonderful with innovative ideas and imagination.

I personally have not had to manage nor imagine the crushing confrontation of the ME disease that my dear friend has had to face.

To have followed what she has gone through, and to see that she has still sustained the energy and determination to be an advocate for acknowledging that this condition exists, and that there is a treatment for it, is incredible and outstanding - I think she is absolutely one of the most incredible women I have ever met.

Samantha Forrest - Lyric Soprano, Opera Singer and Vocal Coach and The American School in Switzerland Performing Arts Department Chair, Montagnola, Lugano, Switzerland.

There we were, a perfect row of uniformed waiting staff, standing shoulder to shoulder in a long line of sea green. We looked like a giant had projectile sneezed across the London Marriott Hotel entrance hall. One by one, Mr Marriott was greeted by the excited nodding puppets, as he made his way down the line, rather like a wedding greeting, but without the bride, or cake! It was Mr Marriot's son officially, but we were instructed to greet him like royalty.

"Good afternoon, Mr Marriott," the row of snot parroted one by one, with a handshake.

Mr Marriott stood opposite me, and with a huge smile he extended his royal hand towards me with "Good afternoon!"

"Hiya love! Are you alright?" I replied in a purposeful broad Lancashire accent and added a cheeky smile. I could feel the maître d' wincing and melting, like the wicked witch she was.

Mr Marriott suddenly froze rigid from his religious greeting pattern and looked down at me, which wasn't uncommon. He burst out laughing at my retort, and I liked him instantly! He proceeded to stay and engage in a light conversation with me for a few minutes, asking where exactly I was from, as my accent had surprised him. He said to the staff, "I like her!" Before hurriedly making his way to the finish line! The maître d' let me keep my own tips that night instead of stealing them, which made me happy, because I had a London rent to cover, and my wages were not nearly enough to survive.

Catching a tube at 2am after being locked inside the hotel fridge freezer on a nightly basis, whilst waiting for someone to rescue me, became a routine event. My featherweight body and short stature wasn't broad or long enough to carry a large, loaded metal tray of cakes in one hand, whilst holding the heavy iron fridge door open with the opposing leg. I would hear the handleless prison cell door bolt shut behind me, and wonder how many cakes I could get through before I froze to death!

With an 8am morning shift, and a two-hour round-trip tube journey, I often wondered if I would get more sleep staying inside the fridge. Now in my early twenties, it was becoming increasingly frustrating that I would frequently feel lightheaded and sick, and at worse, lose my balance and fall over, even more distressing for a dancer to whom balance was essential.

One afternoon, I greeted a beautifully dressed couple into the Marriott hotel dining area with, "Wow you look beautiful. Have you been anywhere nice?" The lady smiled proudly, as she removed her coat, and replied "Yes, we have just been to see the Queen!"

I showed the happy couple to a settee in the corner and took their drinks order. Moments later, smiling broadly with my head held high, I returned balancing a pint of beer and a glass of wine on a circular silver edged tray. As I stepped down the carpeted stair, into the lounge from the adjoining bar area, I suddenly felt dizzy and lightheaded. There was a whirring sound inside my head, as frequently happened. I lost my balance, and the tray tipped forwards spilling the entire contents of the beer all over the poor, now sodden, suited male guest.

Horrified, I apologised unreservedly and immediately moved to his aid, handing him my crisp white napkin and upturning the remaining glasses on the tray, before rushing to the kitchen to get the guest further support. I was reprimanded in the kitchen for my accidental actions, and ordered by the maître d' to "Stay away from these guests!" I had no idea why, as it was a pure accident.

Moments later, I was escorted back into the lounge, and the two guests were very welcoming of me and laughing at the entire event. The man had personally requested my company, and told me that I was "highly entertaining and a lively northerner.", and that he wanted me to look after him and his wife, for the duration of their stay.

It was much later that day, that I found out that the man was football legend; Bobby Charlton, with his wife...which explained why they had told me that they had just been to see the Queen! As a football legend, with one of the most powerful shots in the game, I was thankful that he didn't give me the boot!

I had trained in silver service working as a waitress from the age of sixteen years, firstly at the Barton Grange Hotel in Preston, and then moved to work with my friends, Louisa Cornall and Stephen Pettinger, at The Broughton Park Hotel, Preston, (now The Marriott Hotel).

Silver service was a challenge for anyone petite who lacked strength and balance...well for me!

Carrying heavy silver trays stacked high with hot plates along my short hyper-mobile left arm, and then using a large silver fork and spoon in the right hand, to serve rows of seated guests' hot food, without dropping anything on their lap, was nigh on impossible!

My worst recollection, aside from wetting the head of football stars, was accidentally upturning a hot bowl of tomato soup on an unsuspecting bride's lap. I was horrified and apologetic, as I had taken the hit too, but thankfully she forgave me and laughed, and I realised that this is precisely why alcohol is essential at the top table. I thoroughly enjoyed serving people, and this all helped build self-confidence, later used on stage in stand-up comedy, when bantering with the audience. At university, I had worked at The Roehampton Club, in Surrey, which I recall required a formal audition process to be employed there. Fortunately, whilst working there, I managed to serve Tennis Legend, Goran Ivanišević a bowl of strawberries and cream, without throwing them on him.

I juggled treading the boards in the day, and working as a waitress and a stand-up comedian by night. I figured that as I was getting laughed at in a leotard by day, I may as well get laughed at in a career of comedy, by choice. In desperation to appear taller for my auditions, I was advised by a fellow dancer to invest in some Buffalo Boots. 'The Spice Girls' were regularly featured wearing these fashionable 1990's boots, which had a very high flat platform base.

I was only earning minimum wage, and with a high London rental on my flat, how on earth was I meant to afford a pair of these expensive boots? A rotund, suited gentleman was seated at the end of the London Marriott hotel bar. He had been watching me all night long, racing around the tables, serving customers and excitedly chatting. Shattered, with brown tousled hair sticking to my face from the heat of the kitchen, I stood momentarily by the bar to catch my breath, and wipe away the sweat from my brow.

"Hey! I hear you are a singer."

I looked around and carried on about my business. It was that time of night when the drunks at the bar started hitting on anyone wearing a skirt. Just ignore him.

"Hey don't ignore me. I have got something for you."

I looked over as he held up a crisp £50 note. I had never seen a fifty-pound note before; it didn't look real. It was more than I made on a full day's work shift.

"It is yours if you sing me a song, beautiful!"

Oh blimey. I certainly needed the money. Was this prostitution? I desperately wanted those Buffalo Boots. Egged on by the bar tender, who had manipulated this event, I walked with the gentleman out of the restaurant, and positioned myself ahead of the quiet hotel lobby, and sang one verse of a song.

"That's your lot or I may get fired for not working," I concluded.

The man smiled and handed over the crisp £50 note. "I didn't think you'd do it. You're brave and you have a beautiful singing voice, this money is yours, just as I promised."

"Thank you," I took the cash gratefully, feeling incredibly embarrassed, and hid it inside the top of my shirt. Yes, this certainly felt like prostitution!

I hurried away into the kitchen and finished my night shift promptly. With tonight's hard and easy earned cash, I could now afford those £90 Buffalo Boots. The most expensive footwear I had ever bought!

The following week, I arrive at the dance studio wearing my brand-new boots, auditioning for a musical production, and I was so pleased to find myself dancing on the front line with my childhood friend from Preston, Carolyn Bolton/Kidman Beeson. Carolyn and I danced our hearts out, and we were both lucky enough to get through a number of dance recalls throughout the day.

Used to hearing the casting director's numerical judgement call between each rigorous dance routine, "Number seven, number twenty-three and number sixty-four stay behind!" we were genuinely excited for each other that our numbers were both being called out each time, and as excitable northerners we had lots of news to catch up on over lunch!

By the day's end, exhausted from the adrenaline rush of a combination of dancing and nervous anticipation, we were both recalled to a different audition room to sing. Suddenly alone, I walked with trepidation into a darkly lit room, wearing a huge, outwardly confident smile into the final judgment room, to meet the director, who invited me to perform a song. I finished my solo, and he paused momentarily, looking me up and down, and without any emotion said, "Take your shoes off!"

I followed his instruction without question, and now suddenly two inches shorter, I smiled broadly, holding the heavy black boots with trailing laces, by my sides. There was a long dramatic pause, and I hoped that my huge smile had warmed his heart, particularly after a long gruelling audition day of recalls. I hoped that I had done enough to get through…

"Go home! You've wasted my time!" he snapped.

And that was that.

My new £90 Buffalo Boots had let me down. The director had sent me home, because I was too short. He told me that I wouldn't fit the costume. During the Autumn of 1997, I applied for a waitress position elsewhere, and was really happy to be employed at 'Capital Cafe' in London's Leicester Square.

I thoroughly enjoyed working here, alongside happy, upbeat, enthusiastic, life-long friends from all around the world, working within a fun-filled environment, complete with a central DJ booth and flashing lights, pumping out hit tunes, as we waited on.

My friends included Chanel Miller and Erica Bruce, who both made me feel so welcome, and helped me study to pass my food and beverage examination, where I learned precisely what was inside every single item on the menu, and also how to make cocktails. I felt like Tom Cruise, but without the balance required to carry a tray, never mind juggle glass bottles.

Years later, all these waitressing skills came in useful, as I was employed throughout the UK, as a 'Singing Waiter' and a 'Comedy Waiter', with my very talented vocalist friend, Mark Tedin. Mark and I worked as 'Singing Waiters' at The Marriot Hotel, Bournemouth conference room, for a 'Chiropractic Convention', and after waiting on the formerly suited guests, we would unsuspectingly pick up our hidden microphones from opposite ends of the large conference room, and start singing, in harmonising 'The Prayer' by Celine Dion and Andrea Bocelli.

The reactions from the guests were priceless, as we were dressed as waiters, they would whisper and question if we were meant to be doing this? By the end of the set, the applause was rewarding. One evening, at the Savoy Hotel in Blackpool, Mark and I were booked this time as both 'Comedy and Singing Waiters'.

The large banqueting suite was filled with circular tables, covered in crisp white table covers, and the Army Captains' guests of men and women, seated respectfully around them. Here, Mark and I were instructed by the event bookers, to improvise the performance, 'by dropping things and spilling food on guests' (they had clearly read my C.V.), then we were to have a huge row with each other, before breaking into song. In order for this to work, no one, except the hotel manager, and the Captain knew this was an actual performance.

Prone to laughter, predominantly at my vocal harmonies, Mark was absolutely exceptional in his acting skills and remained in character throughout. Not only did Mark convince the hotel staff and audience that we were both boyfriend and girlfriend, he also managed to convince the whole room that he was straight. We had never fallen out, so this in itself was going to be a challenge.

"We have extra waiting staff working tonight, as it's a big event, so please make them feel welcome," the hotel manager briefed the regular team of waiters.

"My girlfriend and I are having relationship issues," Mark purposely confided loudly to the staff in the kitchen, whilst collecting hot plates to serve the guests. In character, I proceeded to overtly flirt with all the men in the room. Safely knowing that one guest was in on the jokes, I unabashedly sat on the Captain's knee, whilst topping up his red wine. The Captain was laughing at the scene, as Mark walked past in a huff shouting, "Oh Cathy, I cannot believe you are throwing our relationship away like this!"

"Look at her. I'd be fired for that!" exclaimed one of the waitresses, walking past me, and understandably siding with my stage boyfriend, Mark.

I couldn't believe how overtly obvious I was being, and yet everyone in the room was falling for it. I was given a huge smile and a nod of amusement from the hotel manager. The tension in the room continued to build, as Mark and I completed comedy stage trips and falls over the carpet, with water jugs being emptied on guests, and still no one was suspecting foul play.

Mark left the room a few times to laugh and compose himself, as his fan base, particularly amongst the hotel waiting staff had maximised, casting myself as the flirtatious cheating villain! The kitchen was filled with rage at my inappropriate behaviour.

Mark swung back the kitchen door and bellowed, "Cathy! You are my girlfriend and you are cheating on me!"

"I am just having fun, Mark! There's nothing wrong with a bit of fun," I shouted back, ensuring every guest could hear me.

The chit chat and clinking glasses in the room suddenly stopped, and all eyes were on us. Mark gave me the nod for our performance finale. "It's over, Mark. We are breaking up!" I shouted, as I threw a jug of cold water over him. The room was aghast, followed by a deathly silence from inebriated, agitated guests, who were watching a pair of waiters having a relationship tiff at their Christmas Party. We picked up our microphones and Mark confidently announced to the room, "Happy Christmas everyone! Cathy and I are your entertainment this evening. We are your Comedy Singing Waiters booked by your Captain sat over there," as he gestured to the Captain's table.

The Captain's face was beaming with gratitude as he clapped, and the room gradually came alive again and started laughing. Mark and I then broke into song, giving the room an hour-long performance of upbeat party tracks, inviting everyone to the dance floor, of which they willingly participated, thoroughly enjoying their evening.

Whilst packing up our PA system, Mark and I expressed how *real* the illusion of our theatrical performance felt, and we both vowed to never fall out with each other in reality. A number of very confused waiting staff refused to say goodbye to me, whilst hugging Mark, which had us both in hysterics all the way home.

> *"I had the privilege of working with Cathy at Capital Radio Cafe, based on Leicester Square London. I found Cathy enthusiastic and very hard working.*
> *Cathy always had a smile irrespective of hard work and late hours - at times doing double shifts lasting up to fourteen hours on her feet. Her infectious personality and encouraging spirit were unforgettable and played an integral role in lifting the spirit of our team. Forever missed and always remembered - what a gal!"*
> **Chanel Miller - Director/Owner GREENOCK MANOR LLC - Orange County, Virginia, USA**

CHAPTER FIFTEEN: Oh no it isn't ME
It's Behind You!

"I don't like to act because my life is a pantomime anyway." - Karl Lagerfield.

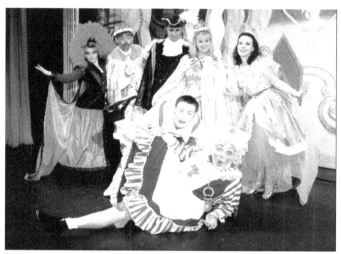

Catherine Vandome as 'Fairy Sunbeam' in 'Sleeping Beauty' with Keith 'Appy' Hopkins as the 'Dame', and Gail Watts as 'Carabosse', at The Princess Theatre, Hunstanton, in Norfolk, in 1998.

"In 1998 I had the privilege of presenting, directing and starring in 'Sleeping Beauty' at The Princess Theatre, Hunstanton, Norfolk. With such a heavy work load I surrounded myself with the best, hard-working talent I could find. That's when I discovered Cathy, and gave her the part of 'Fairy Sunbeam', and what a sunbeam she turned out to be. She gave an outstanding performance every day for the four week, twice daily season."
Keith Hopkins - Actor

"Ooh Dick! I didn't know you were behind me!"

I deliver my line with as much sauciness as I can muster, making my 'Princess Alice' pantomime character more of a cheeky Barbara Windsor 'Carry On' part, rather than a stereotypical innocent princess. As I look out at today's audience, I instantly regret my acting enthusiasm!

Resounding laughter from the audience fills the cold dark steel room. I take in a sea of grey from the all-male presence seated on plastic chairs ahead.

This is the first time I have ever been inside a prison. Apart from one other cast member, I am the only female in the room, and I shiver nervously as one of the audience winks at me, and I instantly know what he's in here for!

I was glad to switch roles to Dick Whittington's 'cat' in the following scene, hiding inside a huge circular grey cat head, with an oversized painted pink grin, and a furry grey skin costume, complete with a large matching grey tail, which I precariously draped over my right arm, as I shuffled around.

All in grey, with a huge beaming smile, I feel like I fit in as one of the inmates. After set breakdown, and a white van drive through central London with the cast, the second of today's three pantomimes is in a local London school.

Here, an inquisitive eight-year-old boy charges the stage, hits me hard on my cat head and then rips the head off me, whilst proudly, and in fairness 'accurately', announces loudly to the room, "It's Alice!"

The rest of the afternoon was even more of a headache.

The third pantomime of the day was in a pub, and the drunken heckles from the few locals paying any attention, encouraged me to banter and go off script to keep my own sanity.

Today's performances were for murderers, violent children and drunks, and they say 'acting is easy.'

Exhausted and sickly, from a 6am start, with yet another bout of tonsillitis, I help break down the set and load it into the van for the final time today, before making my way to the nearest London tube station to travel home.

At around 1am, I start walking home from Neasden tube station to my flat, when I am grabbed from behind and pulled backwards onto the ground into a garden, by a man ordering me to, "Get down and keep quiet!"

I freeze as his arms wrap tightly around me, and I bury my head. In total compliance, I don't make a sound. A few minutes pass and the young man stands up and lets me go.

"I'm sorry for grabbing you. I watched you walking from the station and there was a man pointing a gun at your back as you walked. He started to run towards you, so I grabbed you, but I have just seen him chasing another man across the street, so he was after him not you. This is a dangerous road; you shouldn't be walking down here alone at this hour."

I quizzically thank him, and as I look ahead, I see a man in dark clothes in the distance running. I feel like I am in a James Bond movie. I hurriedly walk back to my flat, feeling as cold as the winter night air, and I wish that I was Miss Money Penny, instead of Miss Money Penniless.

At twenty-four years of age, I receive a letter and a phone call telling me to go straight to the hospital immediately for a colposcopy, following the results of a routine smear test. I am told that I have suspicious cells, likely pre-cancer cells, and the quicker they are removed the better my prognosis.

I stand up post-op, wishing to put this undignified experience behind me and just as in my auditions, I reply, "Thank you for today, I am grateful that you have taken the time to see me!"

"Could Cathy Vandome make her way onto the ice."

The overhead Tannoy fills the London arena, and I look quizzically at my ex-boyfriend as he smiles gleefully at my birthday surprise. The London Knights Ice Hockey Super league have just left the ice, as a small northern girl is about to become the half-time entertainment. I make my way down onto the ice to the sound of deafening music, as the packed arena cheers loudly and I am handed a large pair of black ice skates, and a large brown hockey stick, which is bigger than me. As I quickly fasten my laces, I notice my competitor is a lady twice my height and build, and I immediately shake her hand and introduce myself.

The referee speaks to us as though we are the actual London Knights standard championship players, and he sets up the game for us to play out.

There are two large hockey goals, and a number of strategically positioned orange cones on the ice, and on the referee's instruction we are to skate around the cones, and the first one to complete the assault course and score three consecutive goal wins. I am grateful for my high school hockey training and ice-skating practise, needed to perform in this competition, of which I had absolutely no prior warning. Caught up in the euphoria of the experience with the biggest audience I had ever had, I only half listen to the instructions, as I am so keen to start. Unlike at primary school, I didn't have my best friend Jennifer Woodburn to relay the instructions to my mother, before I began.

"Contenders ready!" or words to that effect, as the referee starts the game.

BEEP!

A loud siren is sounded and we both start to race against each other as per our instructions.

I whizz past the lady, controlling my puck with the hockey stick and weaving around the cones at speed.

SLAM!

I score my first goal, as my competitor is giggling and slipping on the ice, and not taking this game as seriously as I am.

SLAM!

My second puck is hit straight into the centre back of the netted goal, as I dart past my competitor.

SLAM!

CHEER!!!!

The audience rises to their feet cheering and performing a Mexican wave as I score my third goal, and I drink in the excitement of my surroundings.

We wait patiently for my competitor to score her second goal, and then her third, and we all applaud when she completes the game.

The bemused referee celebrates my win by holding up my right arm to a resounding cheer from the crowd, but he then starts laughing and explains to the audience down the microphone that this has never happened before as, "Cathy has won the competition, but she has accidentally scored into the wrong goals."

This brings much laughter from us all, and I point to my competitor to celebrate her win, as we are the tortoise and the hare, and she has won by default.

The crowd were very kindly cheering in support of me after my sporting efforts, and it was thus decided that we would both win a pair of Ray-Ban sunglasses. I laughingly made my way back to my seat, and as I climbed up the steep steps, my friend Susanne Marston called out to me from within the crowd. After all of our comedically tragic experiences together, she was grateful to be a spectator today at my escapades, and laughed and cheered louder than anyone!

Wearing my new ridiculously expensive sunglasses, this whole experience epitomised my belief to always, 'Laugh and the world laughs with you, weep and you weep alone!' I realised that the hockey goal was 'behind me'.

I moved into my new home in 2007, after many months of redecorating both the inside and out. My friend, Cathy Reid, after working all day as a clinic nurse, pulled up to my house in her posh silver sports car, to collect me for our pre-arranged 'Ladies who lunch'. After a long summer's day of painting the interior of my house, helped by my Auntie Joan and Uncle Peter, that afternoon they had taught me the difference between 'stalactites' and 'stalagmites'.

As a first time decorator and a perfectionist, believing that gloss paint was similar to emulsion, I had generously applied at least five coats of thick gloss paint to my upstairs banister, when it suddenly glooped and began to create stalactites; 'T' for top! Shortly afterwards the paint landed on the new downstairs carpet in stalagmites; 'G' for ground. Every day is an education.

My uncle Peter raced upstairs with a propane butane torch and set the banister alight to strip off the layers of paint, as Auntie Joan and I giggled quietly downstairs, catching the drips on an old bed sheet, whilst learning a vocabulary of new words from upstairs!

I had painted so much, that it became a new found passion. I painted the summer house, the garden fences, the garden furniture, the indoor furniture, and even the inside of the garage and its roof. Apparently, all this painting is not usual. Indeed, it was said by my family that, "If you stood still long enough Cathy would paint you."

As my friend, Cathy arrives, I am still high on paint fumes and now wearing a flowing red dress. I hurriedly grabbed my handbag, slipped into my heels, and headed quickly outside to meet her. As fast as lightening, I opened the passenger car door and jumped inside, and amidst my breathless babble, explaining why I was running a little late, I buckled up my seatbelt, and looked forwards through the car window, awaiting a reply.

Silence.

"Cathy, are you there?" I joked, rummaging through my handbag.

"Cathy, are we not setting off?"

Silence

"Cathy!" I giggled, and turned to look at the driver. This was not Cathy. This was a large set man, a complete stranger, now eerily staring back at me.

"Argh!" I cried, whilst frantically unbuckling my seat belt in a rush to exit the vehicle.

The man said nothing. Just watched me. I looked behind me, and Cathy was seated in her car behind this one, laughing uncontrollably.

"I wondered what you were doing!" she giggled, as I scrambled into her car.

"Oh blimey! That was a stranger, he could have driven off with me!" I panted.

"I know! I've been sat here, behind you!" Cathy laughed, as she turned on the ignition.

"Worse still, he could have thought, 'Well I didn't pay for this, but she will have to do!'"

This fuelled much resounding laughter from us both, for our usual comedy filled dinner ahead.

The steep hill-climb, once more, forces me to change down to second gear, as I take in the breathtaking scenic views of the surrounding countryside, either side of the never-ending rolling road. My feet are tightly strapped into the pedals of my silver mountain bike, enabling greater power, as I push my body to the max on the biggest physical exercise challenge I have endured, and incorporating just one rest stop.

Cycling from Guildford to Brighton, on today's challenge with my ex-boyfriend, I am red faced, bleary eyed and open mouthed. I gasp for air through constricted lungs, and question how on earth I will make it all the way to the seaside. As I slide into fourth gear, the road ahead finally becomes linear.

I unhook my tired feet from the black pedal straps, and rest them atop the pedals, as I whirr down Brighton seafront, grateful for the end of a vertical hill climb and the opportunity to free-fall to the finish line. I wish my black silicone gel padded cycle seat had been as effective as it was guaranteed in the cycle shop!

I glide gently towards the last approaching seafront hotel on my left, opposite the beach with the bright gold rotating carousel ride, now filling the air with the sound of organ bells, when I feel my bike jolt backwards to a sudden stop, and I am flown sideways onto the pavement with a 'thud'.

Male voices and high-pitched laughter fill the evening air, and I notice a group of young teenage boys pointing; they had pulled my bike pannier backwards for a cheap laugh. They did not know that I had just cycled the best part of sixty miles, on a challenging hill route, and though I was grateful for a lie down, the dramatic dismount had ruined my celebratory finish!

As I attempted to stand up, it was as though cement had filled my entire bruised body. I could barely take a step, never mind drag a large mountain bike.

"This is strange, my legs are so heavy they won't walk," I told my ex-boyfriend, who came to my aid.

Despite minor aches and pains, my ex-boyfriend was able to walk fine, but I strangely could barely move, and the following day, as I shuffled to the train station with heavy lead legs, he cycled easily back home.

BANG!

I jolt forcefully forwards and backwards inside my car, following an emergency stop, gripping the steering wheel tightly with both hands, whilst questioning what on earth has just happened?

I am shaken up, and frozen to my seat with fear.

A gentleman wearing red appears at my driver side window, and opens the car door to check on me.

I notice his red van, and in my sudden confusion, I think he's an ambulance driver and that they are now uniformed in red, which would of course make more practical sense!

"I saw everything," the man panted, having raced out of his van. "I am your witness."

The man explained that I had just been a victim of a purposeful attempted crash, and that the perpetrator had indicated left and started turning into my road, and then intentionally, suddenly changed direction and sped up in attempt to hit me, as I was turning right. Luckily, I was turning out slowly, and I managed to slam on my brakes. The car had continued forwards and crashed into a huge tree, and both the driver and the passenger were not wearing seatbelts, for maximum compensation claim injuries.

As the police and ambulances arrived, the man advised me to go straight to hospital inside the ambulance, and get myself checked out. I was deathly white; he hadn't realised that was my natural complexion. Once inside the hospital, the consultant was talking to me, following his assessment, which found that my back, neck, right arm, and shoulder had taken the brunt of the whiplash, and now that the adrenaline had stopped, I was feeling a lot more pain.

Suddenly, the green cubicle curtain whipped open, and an apologetic police officer said that he needed to speak to me immediately. I was thankful that he hadn't timed that five minutes sooner!

The officer took a statement from me, and I thought that this was a very unusual occurrence. He asked me if anyone at the crash site or inside the hospital had suggested a motorbike was present at the scene?

"Yes," I replied. "Here in the hospital, a concerned family gathered around me earlier, and they asked me whether I had seen a motorbike at the crash site, and I told them that I hadn't."

"They are criminals, Catherine. You're not the first victim; they're making up a false witness on a motorbike to support themselves."

I felt as though I was inside my own television crime series. I was expecting Nick Ross to appear next! The police were completely behind me, and sometime later the offenders were prosecuted. I spent a week in bed in chronic pain, and with time to reflect, I realised the pantomime scriptwriters were right - they were all indeed "behind me!"

A most memorable and defining moment in my theatrical career came in 1998, aged twenty-four years, when I auditioned for Barrie Stacey and Keith Hopkins, at Ronnie Trafford/Parnell Productions in London's West End.

Barrie Stacey became my Musical Theatre Agent and provided me with incredible career opportunities.

I was so grateful to be cast as 'Fairy Sunbeam' in 'Sleeping Beauty' at The Princess Theatre in Hunstanton, Norfolk, with the talented actress Gail Watts as the evil 'Carabosse', and alongside the brilliantly gifted Keith Hopkins as the 'Dame'. I would soon discover that I had previously performed with Keith Hopkins, as a young dancer, in the Trafford/Parnell Productions UK Tour of 'The Wizard of Oz' at Preston's Charter Theatre. It was an absolute joy and an honour to work with both of the West End legends, Barrie Stacey and Keith 'Appy' Hopkins.

"If pantomime success is measured in decibels, 'Sleeping Beauty is a roaring hit - and we don't need an invitation to join in, we are cheering Fairy Sunbeam, engagingly played by Catherine Vandome."
'The Stage' review January 1998 - Sleeping Beauty.

"It is no surprise that Hopkins' loyal following has made this a record-breaking box office hit at The Princess."
Alison Croose - local review 1998.

"Very fond memories of a panto cast that became a Christmas family, the year Hunstanton snow stopped us all going home!
The crazy loveable fairy, Cathy Vandome to my evil Carabosse, was an experience I will treasure…very fond memories of one of our days off, when we all bundled into my Land Rover and drove to Sandringham gardens to get a glimpse of royalty whilst having crazy snowball fights…and after twenty-one years we have managed to hold onto the friendship that came from 'Sleeping Beauty' madness. Love and hugs chickadee xxx"
Gail Watts – Actress

After completing a winter season in Hunstanton, I auditioned again in 1999 for Barrie Stacey and I was cast as 'Kaa' the snake in 'The Jungle Book' performing at The Wimbledon Theatre in London.

"Catherine Vandome played the part of Kaa the snake in my production of 'The Jungle Book'. The show toured all over the country for many years. I, and the company, was never the same again, and neither was the jungle! Catherine brought such energy to the part. Well done and many thanks!"
Barrie Stacey - West End Theatrical Agent from 1972, and Author of 'A ticket to the Carnival', which sees Barrie unravel his decades as a performer, agent, producer and impresario. Cherished U.K. thespian Barrie Stacey has shared the stage with Quentin Crisp and Frankie Howerd, Jessie Matthews, Russell Grant and Diana Dors. Barrie is recently deceased at aged 95 years (1926-2022).

CHAPTER SIXTEEN: Entertain ME!
'Best' of times!

"I'll have what she's having." - When Harry Met Sally, 1989.

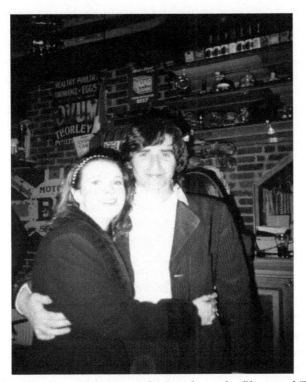

Catherine Vandome with Actor John Lynch, on the film set of 'Best', in Ireland, in 1999.

Blessed are the cracked for they shall let in the light" - Groucho Marks.
Never did a phrase describe a person with such a poignant meaning; a simple truth.
Cathy entered the room and the room filled with light, and I remember that very clearly, despite the geography, and the room still fills with light to this day.
We became fast friends, as Cathy's addictive personality can not only fill a room full of atmosphere, her presence changes the air, the temperature, the conversation.
Switching between self-deprecating jokes, to a passionate study of your life and the people within it, a conversation is never a boring experience, as small talk is an unfathomable idea for Cathy. A far more ridiculous and often hilarious chit chat is delivered.

My memories are filled with this quintessential notion which sits alongside my understanding of her character - Cathy as a caring, loving woman, who's strength and heart has carried her through the best and hardest of times.

I was so happy when we met professionally on film. a biography about George Best and who should turn up, that's right, Ms Catherine Vandome... and the set filled with light. The cast and crew fell in love with her.

We were shooting on location, and I seem to remember her part was shot over three days, but she stayed the week.

Every time I turned around, she was chatting to someone: the Script Supervisor, an electrician, the caterer, the Prop Master and at one point she had one of our cast members in tears of laughter. That wit and the gift of fast chit chat has never left her.

When we were together on set, I think everyone was so happy because she was there, particularly in the evenings, as we were all away from home, and from our friends and our families. So, a night out with Cathy seemed to lift everyone's spirits, particularly when she jumped onto a drum set at a nightclub, and played a set out with a local band. That poor drummer never got a look in.

Her character has been a constant inspiration in my life. Despite her illness, nothing has stopped her from fulfilling her dreams, and that is because she has an inner strength that comes from her heart, and from that her light shines through with warmth, love and of course the most important thing - laughter.

Work Colleague - 'Best'

In 1999, I travelled to Northern Ireland to film a small part in the film 'Best.'

'Best' was about the life and football career of the Northern Irish football star, George Best. It was directed by Mary McGuckian and starred John Lynch as the late George Best. The film premiered on 1st May 2000. I arrived in Ireland, and stayed in a hotel and I was welcomed by such a wonderful cast and crew, that the joy and laughter continued into the small hours. Working in film was great fun, and a different experience to what I had been used to throughout my career in live theatre. Primarily being, that if you make a mistake, you can start again. I learned a lot from watching the cast and crew at work,

The very talented actor John Lynch, playing the staring-role of 'George Best' in the movie, was such a kind-hearted gentleman, and a true professional in his field. George Best himself, came into the bar as we were filming, and fortunately for him I wasn't working as a waitress, so thankfully I didn't manage a hat trick and spill a pint down this footballing legend!

In order to be available for auditions, I worked numerous promotional jobs as a model, presenter and a make-up artist, for many large events, both UK and worldwide, including the London Ideal Home Exhibition, The Birmingham Motor Show, Royal Ascot, and The Clothes Show.

In between auditions, I would work enthusiastically, often ten-hour days, promoting and selling a wide range of company promotional products. One day I would be modelling on top of a Ferrari with Michael Schumacher, and the next selling hundred-pound toothbrushes in my hometown of Preston, where I somehow managed to win the UK top sales of toothbrushes, which was a complete surprise, as most people in Preston don't brush their teeth!

Always up for a challenge, I would promote and sell almost anything and everything, including The Tanning Shop treatments, where passers-by in Kensington, on collecting my fliers, would point and laugh at my 'Adams' family' complexion, and say, "Well it clearly doesn't work!", and my personal favourite was modelling for a brand-new hairdresser's salon, where I arrived asking for a 'Rachel' from 'Friends' haircut, and left as 'Rose West'.

The only thing I couldn't do prior to the event promotions was to blow up a balloon. A simple task to many, but an impossible task for me. Rather like the impossibility of cartwheeling leading with my right arm, as I can only cartwheel on my left side, but even worse, because unlike normal people, I somehow didn't have enough puff to blow up a balloon. When I tried to blow up a balloon, with much surrounding laughter from the other models, I would afterwards pass out, before the Event Manager took me seriously. I had so many left over free samples of hair and beauty products and food and beverages, that I would give them to my nana back home in Preston, to see the excitement on her face.

Nana would excitedly stock up her little box room with boxes of cereal and laugh, "Eeh Cathy! If we have another war, we won't go hungry!"

"No Smint no kiss!" I said bravely puckering up to the television newsreader Trevor McDonald, as I walked up to him over London Bridge. He looked down at a small northern lady, dragging a trolley full of Smint mints, and dutifully declined the offer of either the mint, or the kiss.

In 1999, I appeared in 'The Stage' newspaper as a make-up artist and in the same year, I was booked on a U.K. Tour of 'Back to our Roots' with T.V. personalities 'Mel and Sue', Melanie Giedroyc and Sue Perkins. I was Mel and Sue's personal make-up artist, and watching the very talented duo perform, increased my desire to want to work as a stand-up comedian.

We all enjoyed every minute of the tour, which was filled with lots of laughter, amidst the long hours of daily travel to each of the theatre venues.

Mel and Sue are absolutely wonderful artists and genuine kind-hearted people, and they gave me great insight both behind the scenes, and on stage, into the art of performing live stand-up comedy.

They both welcomed me into the tour, and made me feel like an integral part of the production family, allowing me to play the drums on stage a number of times, during the pre-show warm up jamming sessions with the band.

Backstage, Mel and Sue introduced me to their friends and incredibly talented stand-up comedians, Dawn French and Jennifer Saunders, and Bob Downe. This invaluable learning opportunity from many of the best entertainers in comedy, helped to later pave the way into my own career in stand- up comedy.

The following year, I toured the UK and Ireland as a Presenter for L'Oreal and for Boots UK, opening business conferences and fashion shows, and using an auto-cue. However, one morning, I arrived at a job in London with the 'brief' being literally to model for a lingerie company. As I walked into the studio a number of the models were arguing, and some had started to leave the building, sounding distressed.

I was led to believe by the agency that I would be wearing a t-shirt and shorts and modelling indoors, for a commercial shoot. However, I was thrust a black pair of knickers (the size of a tea bag), with a smaller sized black bra displaying a tiny product company logo the size of a thumb nail, topped with a beige flasher mack. I was grouped into a mix of five boys and girls. The boys were costumed in appropriately styled t-shirts and shorts, which more clearly displayed the lingerie product company logo. I was given a set of instructions from the lingerie head office which read;

> "Groups of five models are to travel across London on the underground stations in full costume at all times. In the morning session, models are to position themselves on the allocated station platform seating and as soon as the tube pulls out of the station, models are to jump up and open their flasher macks and flash their pants to the unsuspecting commuters. Please note that should any of the group be arrested by the police, they must simply reply "We are just having a bit of a laugh."
>
> The afternoon session will comprise of all the models together (those who have not been arrested) to march across London's Bond Street and Oxford Street jumping on and off commuter buses sitting next to passengers and flashing your pants at all times. Please note that anyone refusing to flash their pants will not get paid!"

As hilarious as this job was, for all the wrong reasons, that day I decided that there had to be better ways to make my London rent. I was lucky that my ex-boyfriend was working with me this day, but when the team leader repeatedly bellowed down Oxford Street "Flash your pants or you won't get paid!" my ex-boyfriend retorted, "Flash your pants again, Cathy, and you're dumped!" Business mogul Lord Alan Sugar would undoubtedly have felt that the product placement on the female models' costumes, was completely illegible!

> I have worked with Cathy for many years in many different settings, from doing tech for her Sparkle Theatre company, to helping support Cathy at her shows in Holiday Parks, and working-men's clubs up and down the country.
>
> One of my favourite and funniest memories at this time, was when Cathy was performing her '80's Diva Show' and we convinced an extremely attractive man and a vicar to dance with me to the song 'Hot Stuff' by Donna Summer, continually taking off more and more clothes. On one side there was an adonis of a man, and on the other a vicar who was so excited to be on stage, that we almost got him down to his white collar!
>
> But during all of this, there were also times that were worrying and down-right scary. I remember during one of Cathy's gigs, where after performing and entertaining the crowd for over an hour, Cathy came off stage into the small broom closet we were given as a dressing room and collapsed.

This was extremely worrying, especially as this was not the first time of her illness showing. It also just scared me to see a friend so extremely weak. The only thing we could do was to get her some water and give her some time to recover.

I took down all the equipment and packed it into the car, and then afterwards Cathy came out of the dressing room with the audience completely unaware of anything that had happened behind the scenes.

After this Cathy had to stop performing and was eventually diagnosed with ME. During all of this pain over the years, Cathy still found joy and laughter. That's the best thing about Cathy, she always finds a way to laugh, and not only that, she makes you laugh along with her. That is why I'm so proud of her for writing this book and so proud to call her a dear friend.

Joseph Pollard - Entertainer

CHAPTER SEVENTEEN: Audition ME
Drama Queen!

"An audition's an opportunity to have an audience." - Al Pacino.

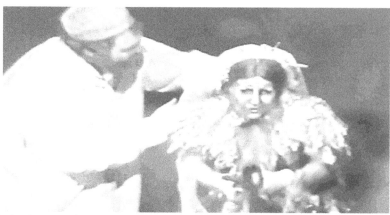

Catherine Vandome as 'Grandma Tzeitel' in 'Fiddler on the Roof' with Daren Blanck as 'Tevye', directed by Gerry Tebbutt, at the Yvonne Arnault Theatre in Guildford, Surrey, in 2000.

I imagine all those, who work in the performing arts industry learn very quickly that tenacity is needed to face rejection, refusal and when things aren't working out in their favour, the need to do something positive.

In the case of Catherine Vandome, she faced the most enormous challenges - far more than anyone I know working in this crazy industry.

Catherine was a student of mine when she attended a Musical Theatre course at the Guildford School of Acting, graduating in 2000.

During that time, I directed her in 'Fiddler on the Roof' and it was obvious throughout her training that she had something to offer the world of entertainment and was determined to follow her chosen career.

But life dealt Catherine a bitter blow when she suffered from ME and carbon monoxide poisoning, which robbed her of the art of walking and talking, and stopped her pursuing and following her dream.

Now years later, Catherine shows us that her training as a performer, and an understanding of the art of storytelling has led to her writing this book, in order that others might benefit from her own personal story.

If we assume that applause and a standing ovation goes to someone, who has opened our minds and enlightened our views, then surely it goes most deservedly to Catherine for her courage and guts in writing this book and sharing her story, in order that it will help others facing similar circumstances.

Gerry Tebbutt - Head of Musical Theatre at the Guildford School of Acting (GSA) (From 1994 - 2011)

As a naïve northerner, Catholic-raised, twenty-three-year-old, I auditioned for a West End Musical called 'Voyeur'. I had absolutely no idea what this musical title meant, prior to my audition, and after a successful recall of my singing audition piece, 'I don't know how to love him' from 'Jesus Christ Superstar', I was invited to speak to the female casting director, seated ahead in the auditorium. The casting director looked me up and down as I sat down next to her. My tight fitted dress and heels, full make up and long brown hair, appeared to have caught her attention. "Congratulations on your singing audition, you have a beautiful singing voice. You are through to the dance auditions at 1pm today."

"Thank you very much." I smiled.

"Just one question," she continued. "You do know that there is nudity in this musical production, don't you? Would you be prepared to take your clothes off?"

"Err…" I choked on my plastic bottle of water.

Not wanting to appear ungrateful for the opportunity, or super naive, which was of course exactly how I looked, I inhaled and relied heavily on my acting training.

"Of course not. That is absolutely fine!… Er.. what kind of nudity?" I confidently replied.

"Full nudity."

Complete shock and silence.

"No problem at all," I lied with a confident smile.

My mind raced, as I left the auditorium, and like the sheep I was, I joined the rest of the herd next door for the dance auditions. I remembered joking with an acting agent, once saying "I don't do nudity. Mind you, they'd probably pay me to keep my clothes on!"

I was still confused as to what this musical was about, as the afternoon's explicit contemporary dance style choreography ended with me positioned open legged, with my backside in the air, and my hands open cupped between my legs in an 'opened flower' gesticulation. I was lucky that my talented actor friend Allan Osborne was with me that day, and once we were safely back home, he educated me on what 'Voyeur' actually meant, and how there was, "No way that I was ever doing that show", and exactly what the casting director was really expecting from me in that auditorium!

To say that we laughed would be an understatement. I don't think we have ever laughed that much together at what could have been! I later discovered that 'Voyeur' the musical was taken down for explicit sexual obscenity after just a couple of nights, although as a naive northerner, I was grateful to have had the opportunity to have learned a 'new word.' I decided from here on in, only to audition for shows of which I understood the title!

After numerous West End audition recalls, including an audition for 'Les Miserable', where I was recalled by 'Cameron Macintosh's Agency' for the musical 'Cats', I was informed that I would have a much stronger chance of getting through, if I had trained at drama school. I decided to audition for The Guildford School of Acting (G.S.A.), which at the time was ranked the third best drama school in the country, and a place where actors, Michael Ball and Brenda Blethyn had trained. I recalled my drama teacher from the University of Surrey, recommending that I go to drama school, but it was easier said than done!

In 1999, I was invited to the very last week of auditions for that year's intake, and I was asked to dance and sing, as well as perform two contrasting acting speeches, in front of a panel of professionals, including the very talented Head of Musical Theatre, Gerry Tebbutt.

By now, I had previous professional theatre work experience, as well as having had numerous auditions, so although extremely nervous, I enjoyed the audition experience, and put everything I could into it. During the acting audition process, I was asked to read a play script. I was being tested on my speech and reading skills, and that day I learned something very interesting about myself. I was asked if I was dyslexic, because I read a piece of literature aloud incorrectly.

I read, "The mat that the cat sat on," instead of "The cat sat on the mat." I learned that I was reading words on a page so fast, that when I spoke the words aloud, I altered the structure of the sentence. Years ahead, I would learn that ME patients' brains, "Speak fast, think fast and move fast." For now though, I was thoroughly enjoying living my fast paced life! At the Guilford School of Acting, now aged twenty-five, and after being told at age seventeen, that I wasn't good enough to go to drama school, I surprisingly achieved my dream goal.

Here in training, I was blessed to work with many talented international artists on my course, including actor Jamie Beamish, from Ireland, singer Sigriour Eyrun Frioriksdottir from Iceland, and actor Daren Blanck from the U.S. I mentally and physically pushed myself to the maximum, to try to learn as much as I possibly could, in order to try to achieve my musical theatre childhood ambitions.

I lived with a wonderful and very talented musical theatre housemate and friend, Caroline Keiff, and we laughed non-stop, always finding the joy in everything we did, whilst working hard and thoroughly enjoying our time at drama school. Caroline and I would entertain ourselves by watching 'The Vandome family holidays' home movies, in which my talented younger brother David, had cleverly edited them, to make my father Steve, the comic star of every scene. Whether that was of my father swimming underwater and resurfacing to the 'Jaws' theme, or of him strolling innocently down the beach, then edited at the fast speed, to the theme of 'Baywatch.'

Each movie brought increasing laughter to our evenings, and whilst most people reached for a glass of wine, Caroline and I would reach for another of the 'Vandome comedy boxset'. Thankfully, like myself, my father has always been game for a laugh, and thanks to my brother David, he now has a better movie showreel than most acting professionals.

I cycled daily into drama school, and in all weathers, a thirty-minute journey through the centre of the beautiful scenic Guildford town, donned in a black cycle helmet and lycra dance attire, carrying a backpack bursting with ballet and tap shoes, theatre scripts and song lyrics, readily prepared for my 9am opening dance class, tutored by a leading West End performer.

I was fully committed to a day of high physical and mental energetic musical theatre performance workshops, before my return cycle journey home. Every day I smiled broadly, as I cycled past a street comedically named 'Jeffreys Passage'. This had historically been an in-house joke within G.S.A., as students regularly used this as an excuse for being late for class, "Sorry I'm late, I got stuck up Jeffrey's Passage!"

Being late for class was severely frowned upon at G.S.A. and rightly so. Time management skills were absolutely paramount at drama school, in preparation for future castings and auditions.

One of my favourite theatre classes was Stage Combat, which was brilliantly executed and taught by the very talented Andrew Ashenden, who had previously trained at G.S.A.

Stage Combat is unique within the world of performance. An actor in a fight scene must be able to be safe for themselves, their partner(s) and other actors on stage, technical crew (onstage and off) and audience (in making sure that nothing lands on the audience). An actor must maintain the character, say lines and make sure the fight scene is full on intention and energy.

I first met Cathy just before she went to drama school, in a touring pantomime, and then again when she came to drama school. On the two occasions I met Cathy, her very open personality and high physical energy was a very apparent part of her personality.

When Cathy was attending stage combat as part of her training, the physical and mental demands were well within her ability.

Even years later, when I taught Cathy's own drama school students, her drive, enthusiastic nature and physical energy was amazing. Drama training is demanding, being a performer is very demanding, but combining that and running a company and a teaching organisation combined, requires a lot of physical, mental and emotional energy.

Cathy's condition has robbed her of this; her career destroyed because of this, and the drain on who Cathy is as a person is tragic.

ME is an illness that needs to be recognised and have the appropriate treatment to stop other people suffering and losing out the same as Cathy.

Andrew Ashenden - Equity Registered Fight Director, Fight Teacher/Examiner for Actors, Combat Theatrical Training (ACTT) and Chair-person for the Equity Fight Directors' Working party.

Stage Combat is a highly physical sport, and under Andrew's excellent tuition, I learned how to kick and punch and break my opponent's neck, before gouging out their eye. I absolutely loved this new found skill of being able to beat somebody up...without actually hurting them! In one choreographed fight routine, I ran up behind my well-built male opponent Alex Reid (former MMA) mixed martial arts fighter, to break his neck, and I was thrown over his shoulder onto the floor into a backward roll. The routine progressed into armed combat using a rapier, sword and dagger and ended in my dramatic death with a grand finale of Alex gauging out my eye! I loved dying on stage…I was used to it!

One night, my very talented friend, Anna Harcourt and I, decided to utilise these stage combat skills inside the local pub. In stark contrast to our recent musical production performance, where we were scantily clad in basque and suspenders, as we shook and shimmied everything we could, whilst leaving sequins and feathers everywhere, today we were stood afoot of the 'Winford' Pub, where we proceeded to beat each other up…for a laugh!

After multiple clearly staged punches to the left and right eyes, followed by dramatic rolls across the floor and winces in pretend pain, Anna and I were laughing so much that to us, it was obvious that this was acting. Our surrounding group of friends were crying with laughter, into their straw clad drinks. However, as soon as I gave Anna the penultimate 'nose grab', by holding her nose between my forefinger and middle finger, whilst she exaggeratedly jumped up and down like a springy frog on illicit drugs, a bouncer grabbed the back of both our coats, and sternly escorted us out of the pub. "We were just having a bit of a laugh!" I said in our defence, quoting the 'Lingerie modelling' job. "It looked very real to me!" the camp, angry bouncer went on. This brought increased laughter to Anna and I, and our friends soon joined us outside all laughing in hysterics, that anyone would believe that this was actually a real fight.

The next morning on my way to G.S.A. I reflected on how I was now fulfilling everything that I had ever dreamed of doing in my childhood. I was waking up singing, dancing and acting by day, and then getting into pub brawls by night! Life could not get any better than this.

As comical and innocent as my evening had been, Andrew Ashenden rightfully highlighted to the stage combat group why actors must not perform stage fighting routines socially, for health and safety reasons. Perhaps if Anna and I had been wearing our previous show costumes of basques and suspenders, we may have been 'tipped' in the pub, instead of being 'tipped' out of it!

Though incredibly challenging both mentally and physically at G.S.A. I learned *so* much from some of the most highly esteemed professionals in the business, including Gerry Tebbutt, Jill Francis and Tracey Collier, all passing their knowledge and experience on to me, preparing me for the challenging world ahead of musical theatre. My most memorable role was playing 'Grandma Tzeitel' in a musical production of 'Fiddler on the Roof' by Jerry Bock, Joseph Stein, and Sheldon Harnick, masterfully directed by the head of G.S.A. Gerry Tebbutt, and staged at the Yvonne Arnault Theatre, in Guildford. With an ever-mounting C.V. of comedy old ladies including a recent performance of the 'Landlady' in 'Lucky Stiff', by Lynn Aherens and Stephen Flaherty, I was over the moon to be cast as 'Grandma Tzeitel'. However, I found this particular scene in 'Fiddler on the Roof' so terrifying to watch in my childhood, that I now struggled to watch it again, knowing that I was actually going to play the nightmare Grandma character for real!

Somehow, I overcame my fears, and played 'Grandma' with full integrity in mimicking the characterisation of the 'on screen' stooped old lady shuffling along with a walking stick. I tried to add a comedic overtone to the role, whilst playing it for real, exactly the way my drama teacher Carol Buckley had originally taught me to do. I laughed, as I again recalled my high school drama teacher telling me to, "Stop playing old ladies!" Here I was continuing to make a professional career out of it!

My G.S.A. end of year 'Agent Showcase' was performed at The Fortune Theatre, Russell Street in London's West End. The Fortune Theatre is renowned for staging the long running, haunting play 'The Woman in Black'. This longstanding theatre is unique and has a 'raked stage', which means that actors have to literally walk 'upstage' to the back and 'downstage' to the front. Hence where the theatrical terminology originated from, as the original stages were built with raked stages. There is a felt sense to performing on such a historic stage, which is renowned for its nightly 'horror genre' theatrical play. The surroundings, both backstage in the dressing rooms, and inside the auditorium itself, are dark and eerie and it feels icy cold. I am warned backstage, "There is a belief that the theatre itself is haunted, and that 'The Woman in Black' ghost is actually real".

'The Woman in Black' is 'short, thin, deathly white, and has dark hair.' and in the play she is renowned for floating around the auditorium.

Costumed in a pale coloured 1920's dress, and petite heeled shoes, I walk nervously down the raked stage, and perch sideways on the garden bench positioned centre stage. I begin my sketch as 'Doris' from 'My Mother Said I Never Should,' by Charlotte Keatley. (Act 111 scene 8), and I follow this, by singing a comedic rendition of the song 'Bill' from the musical 'Showboat' to my onstage husband, played by the comic actor Ben Woolrych, who sat by my side, enjoying a picnic.

At the end of the piece, I lean forward eyes closed, and pucker up ready to kiss my onstage husband. However, for optimum comical impact, instead of kissing me, I have pre-directed Ben to smile at the audience, and put his half-eaten sandwich into my mouth, as the lights go down.

After everyone has performed their pieces, I am joined by our very talented group of performers, many of whom became industry professionals, and together we conclude the show with a powerful vocal group harmony rendition of the "Opening Sequence: The New World," from the musical, "Songs for a new World," by Jason Robert Brown.

As the curtain comes down, I am over the moon to learn that I am being signed up by a 'West End Theatrical Agent', who has talent spotted me, and taken me on following today's showcase performance. However, looking exactly like the Woman in Black, I am fully aware that the elderly gentleman had likely believed me to be the 'Fortune Theatre's apparition!'

Thinking of a story for you dear Cathy…
Do you recall daring to stand on a glass bottomed balcony of a glass penthouse apartment. I was thinking "Oh what the heck! This is not for the faint hearted, it's a cruel form of vertigo torture!"

You on the other hand unfazed, said what worried you was, "If I were to scratch me botty there's a chance in this 360 degree glass house that someone somewhere may snatch a glimpse they may regret snatching!" ... intake of breath... infectious laughter!

I also recall a cautionary tale once upon a night in the 'Winford.' boozer.

On that particular evening the ambience was punctuated, if not punctured, by us being drag handled out by the door whore, who thought you and I were having a right royal punch up!

Intent was merely to demonstrate a comical stunt fight, and Cathy you are always first willing, darling!

We thought we were having a silly old larf showing off as per usual!... but management were convinced it was genuine and grabbed us by our scruffs and booted us out for having a cat fight in a public bar.

Comedy stage fighting included 'nose twisting', 'hair ripping' and 'head butting'...slamming entertainment was obviously not up their strasse! An unintentional spontaneous floor show! We were spectacular!... and that sums you up dear darling Cathy!

Ps I still have the scar on my left buttock! And you were on lemonade all night and you started it! Love you XX Anna.

Anna Harcourt – Performer and Producer

CHAPTER EIGHTEEN: Laugh with ME
Stand Up for Yourself!

"Laugher is the best medicine." - Proverbs 17.22 of the King James Bible.

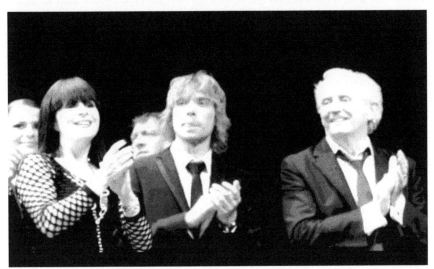

Catherine Vandome performing with Singer and Musician Tony Christie, at the Charter Theatre Preston's 'Big Guild Gig' in 2012.
(Photography: by Jonathan Ince)

I first met Cathy Vandome in 2012 when she did a warmup gig for me, which was very refreshing to see her not only do stand-up comedy, but also a 'Jessie J Tribute' show.
Cathy was energetic, funny and so engaging.
I performed on stage with Cathy at a number of venues over the two years that followed, and was blown away by her ability to never waste a breath, whether it was delivering gags or singing extremely challenging songs, in a way that can only be described as 'dynamic'.
I was saddened to hear that in 2014 she suddenly collapsed very sick and could no longer work alongside me.
Cathy is determined to recover from ME and I have every faith in her tenacity because she is a born performer, and I will certainly be there to help her get back on the stage where she belongs, and as an incentive, I have promised her that she can join me on my planned theatre tour next year.
Lester Crabtree - Comedian and Author of 'Born to Die'

Entertainment venues in the 1980's were always filled with a cloud of cigarette smoke, and the audiences fuelled with alcohol. This was completely normal. Performers would enter the stage within a billow of smog from the dry ice machine, which added to the blanket of cigarette smoke from the punters. To date, live shows are always filled with loud music, flashing lights and toxic chemicals.

The first time I was introduced to stand-up comedy was in 1983, aged nine, at a Pontin's holiday camp. I sat cross legged at the front of a semicircular row of children on the huge ballroom floor, afoot of the adults peering over us, themselves seated on wooden chairs around circular tables lined with multiple alcoholic drinks, atop little white serviettes, with ashtrays spewing cigarette stubs.

Children were not allowed to bring bottles of pop onto the dance floor, so my small fizzy glass of R. Whites Lemonade with a stripy red and white straw, was sat waiting for me centre table, with my parents sat across from each other, eager to have some adult time away from their three children. It was the first time my parents had ever lost track of the time. We had all been so engaged by the 'Hypnotist Act' and were laughing so much at the grown man on the end of the hypnotist line, who ended the show frantically jumping up and down shouting "Mummy, Mummy, I need a wee-wee!"

My elder brother looked at me and we bowed our heads and kept quiet, so that our parents wouldn't remember we were here, and send us to bed. The stand-up comedian tonight was from Wales. All I remember was him walking towards us with a long corded microphone in hand, to a huge round of applause, his opening line ending with "Lay back and Prestatyn!…" , before I felt my father's arms whisk me upwards, as he hurriedly carried me outside to exit the ballroom before his next joke!

I was laughing along with the entire ballroom, and I knew at this moment that I wanted to be just like that old man on stage, and make people laugh for a living! I kept asking my parents what the joke meant, and they said "They didn't know, because they didn't hear it!" A very good Catholic response!

My parents then informed me that Pontins had told them there were to be no more evening cabaret shows scheduled for the remainder of that week. They said "Once Captain Croc had sang 'Goodnight Campers, see you in the morning!' then it was all the children's bedtime!"

It would be four decades later that my good friend and talented stand-up comedian Lester Crabtree would tell me the full joke that I'd missed as a child: "A girl asked me to turn her on by speaking to her in Welsh…so I said ok…Lay back and Prestatyn!"

My first ever stand-up comedy show was at the 'Amused Moose' in Soho, in London's West End, and I was on the same billing as comedy legend, Frank Skinner. It is common for established comics to open a show at one venue, and then close a show at another, as the headline. In doing so, the comic will often try out 'new material' at the first show and mix in a few headline gags, using his 'best material' for the late spot.

That night I followed Frank Skinner immediately after he left the stage, so on my very first night, he was 'unofficially' my warm up act! I was warned that if Frank's material didn't go down well, that I would have a bad night. I couldn't imagine that Frank would ever have a bad gig, and of course he absolutely 'stormed it' and thanks to him lifting the room, I entered the stage to a rapturous applause!

My first ever five minutes of comedy went well, but I knew that this was only the beginning, and that I now had so much to learn. I performed within central London, and throughout the UK as a stand-up comedian, a character comic, within an improvisational comedy group, and as a stand-up comedy club compere.

As a compere, I found that I could use this opportunity to build up my confidence in talking directly to the audience members, and expand beyond the 'stand up material'. My first stand-up comedy show as a compere, was at a prestigious policeman's Ball in Surrey. I was handed a microphone from a fellow comic and told, "Tonight's the night you're going to compere, all you have to do is…talk to them!"

What an adrenaline rush, with no preparation at all and throwing myself in at the deep end.

"Good evening Ladies and Gentlemen…Lock the doors. You're all under arrest!"

As I learned my trade, I was blessed to share the comedy stage over the years, with the very talented comedian Patrick Monahan. Pat is a generous comedian, loved by all who know him, and we had a lot of laughs both on and off stage together, crafting our material. I learned a great deal from him, not only about how to deliver gags, but how to be the best person in life that you can be.

I also performed in many live improvisation comedy shows and I found this the most rewarding. The adrenaline from performing live, on the spot and unrehearsed material was an incredible buzz! A team of three male stand-up comedians and myself, toured London venues with our live improvisation nightly comedy shows. After each performance in three sets, we would always end the show with a 'grand finale'.

"We promised you a human pyramid to conclude tonight's show!" joked the confident compere, who directed the three of us comics, to stand on each other's shoulders. Standing in front of a large glass window of the 'Slug and lettuce' pub, the largest of we three comics, who looked like a friendly bear, braced himself for impact at the bottom of the comedy tower. The next slim built comic, climbed onto his shoulders to an uproar of applause and laugher from the already adrenalized and inebriated crowd.

"And now for the grand finale!" The comic who had confidently opted himself out of this challenge bellowed into his microphone.

A slow clap began, as I successfully climbed up the friendly bear and then continued up to the shoulders of the slim built comic, and without any awareness of my own 'lack of safety' I stood upright at the top of the 'comedy pyramid' and we all balanced perfectly.

Unrehearsed at this death-defying circus feat, we had no idea how to dismount, and so we just sort of fell down like a stack of cards, and somehow, we all survived. The applause was the loudest I had ever heard. Bar staff had frozen aghast at what we had just achieved.

151

The manager offered to buy us all a drink afterwards, and sensibly warned us that it would be best not to attempt this again in front of a large glass window. We didn't just challenge the boundaries of comedy, we challenged the boundaries of health and safety.

The friendly bear was the bravest comedian that I have ever known.

I would often arrive early to the West End comedy venues, and if the bar had been closed all day, it was not uncommon for rats to be scurrying around under the tables. I was like the pied piper of Hamelin, as soon as I started to perform, they all disappeared!

In the early 2000's, most of the stand-up comedy clubs in London's West End were smoking venues. It was six years later, on November 30th 2006, that England and Wales banned smoking indoors. It became my personal plea to stop all smoking in comedy venues, as they were my place of work and passive smoke made me very sick indeed. By now, I had been diagnosed asthmatic, and I am in no doubt that the London smog combined with the nightly cigarette smoke, were a contributing cause.

To try and combat the cigarette smoking inside comedy clubs, I added an 'anti-smoking' comedy song into my new stand-up show, and in time, a newly designated 'Non-smoking Comedy Club' was set up. As I performed my new comedy show, I would invite a 'cigarette smoking man' up onto the stage next to me, whilst he was holding a cigarette. I rewrote the song lyrics to the Karen Carpenter classic, 'Close to You' and I invited my unsuspecting male stooge to sit on a bar stool beside me, whilst I sang to him romantically...

"When you light up a single cigarette, are you aware of the effect? The smoke will rise, and get in your eyes...polluting you... so just like me, girls long to be...Far from You!"

One night at a comedy venue in London's Leicester Square, I was seated on a male stooge's knee singing to him. The audience member was drunk and laughing and loving all of the attention on stage. He helped generate a great comedy room. A successful comedy show is 90% audience and 10% artist. If the audience is on side, it's an easy gig!

At the end of my act, the audience and I gave him the round of applause he deserved, as he made his way back downstairs to refuel at the bar, still laughing loudly!

As I was closing the show, I heard the sound of an ambulance outside, and I said to the audience jokingly, "That bloke's not come back, I think he's laughed himself to death!"

Suddenly, his friend walked up the stairs from the bar, and answered me saying, "My mate was laughing so much that he has fallen down the steep vertical stairs from top to bottom, and has been taken away in an ambulance!"

As I felt responsible for this tragedy, I thought it was only right to have a minute's silence for him, as he had quite literally, "Laughed himself to death." We all agreed that it was the way he would have wanted to go!

It is common for a comedian to die on stage, but not the audience!

One of my first ever stand-up shows in central London was when I died horribly, in fact it was the worst I have ever died, before or since. I was trying out a lot of new material, and quite often it is 'the confidence in the delivery', not the 'material' that does not work. That night I felt nervous, and therefore I looked nervous.

I opened with, "I'm from up north. Growing up we were so poor that my dad used to give me a lift to town on his back."

Maybe a smile.

"I'm so short...I..."

"I feel sorry for you!" a young man heckled.

This is what dying feels like.

I felt sick to the stomach and yet I completed my set, which ended with a cry on a night bus home.

My stand-up comedian friend laughed "You died! Well done! It happens to us all. Now you have absolutely nothing to be afraid of."

I had just lost my stand-up comedy virginity.

I carried on touring the comedy clubs, doing stand-up and comparing shows as myself, and as well as this I also enjoyed dressing up in costumes and creating numerous character comic acts. I was very flattered to be compared to the likes of two of the comedy greats, Caroline Aherne and Victoria Wood. I think it was just because I was 'northern', there's not a lot of Lancashire lasses on the comedy circuit, as so few people can understand us!

In 2002, I began combining my live stand-up comedy shows with T.V. studio recording work. I used my character comedy and ability to do multiple accents, as a voice over artist.

Most memorably, I was in 'Audrey and Friends' the British children's animated television series, which aired on CH 5's 'Milkshake', and was created and directed by David Bennett. I played Audrey's mother 'Valerie', performed in a broad Lancashire accent, and I also played various characters with multiple accents including Liverpudlian, and West Country. The T.V. series ran for 26 episodes, and the show is a mix of 2D and CGI-animation, and it gained a minor cult following in New Zealand where it aired on Prime for several years.

I was a Gadget Mistress for 'Too Much T.V.' as a Television Presenter and Model, and I also modelled for a computer-generated character within a computer game. Yes, I was so small that I could fit inside a computer, no problem!

I performed in a number of T.V. adverts, and I was a featured dancer for 'Seven Seas' Cod liver oil tablets, with voice over by Terry Wogan. Alongside the T.V. advert, I was also a model for 'Seven Seas' Cod liver oil tablets, within a number of magazines, following a photographic shoot. As I was being filmed dancing solo, I was asked by the intrigued Producer of the T.V. advertisement, whether I felt safe dancing and jumping into a stag leap whilst wearing six-inch stilettos? I smiled and replied "Honestly, I feel far safer in heels than in flat shoes, as I wear high heels every day!"

I then laughed that, "I would most likely need a life-time's supply of 'Seven Seas' Cod liver oil tablets, after the pressure I was putting onto all my joints for my art!"

I also worked as a presenter, using an autocue, representing L'Oréal, for 'Boots' U.K. Corporate Event Conferences, which toured throughout the U.K. and Ireland. I thoroughly enjoyed performing in all the varying modalities, but my innermost passion was in making people laugh.

My first love was in stand-up comedy, and I learned that it is much easier to hide behind a stand-up comedy character, than it is to be yourself.

In 2003, with the announced outbreak of SARS, whilst many people were living in a state of fear, I used this situation to create a 'bubbly northern holiday camp entertainment host'.

Wearing a full blonde wig, black rimmed glasses, and a mini skirt, whilst holding a large black clipboard, I opened my stand-up act in a broad Lancashire accent with, "Good evening everybody, I'm Sandra from 'Sunny Adventures in Rural Slovenia'…or for short…SARS!"

Laughter…

Working as a stand-up comedian in London, was very different from working up north. In London's West End, I got to perform to audiences from all over the world, and I can honestly say without any doubt, that I found the American audiences were the best. They were always very enthusiastic and grateful audiences and laughed loudly, and they were so complimentary after the shows. In stark contrast, northerners will tell you exactly what they think of you, not afterwards, but as you are performing, and thus making a good entrance is the most important part of your act!

In a broad Burnley accent the drunk local compare slurs into the mic, "Please welcome 'onta' stage… Kitty Von Deem! Now last night's act was bloody shite, let's hope she's better than that!"

"BOO!" the audience bellow as I walk on stage.

"Good evening, everyone, thank you for the warm welcome, if you enjoy tonight's show my names Catherine Vandome, and if not…its Kitty Von Deem!"

Laugher…

An agent suggested that I set up a tribute act and combine singing with stand-up comedy, and so I created a 'Jessie J Tribute Act'.

Backstage, whilst changing into my 'Jessie J Tribute' costume, my friend Nichola knocks on the changing room door to offer preshow support. I say 'changing room' in the loosest possible terms… she knocks on the toilet door.

"Cathy, I thought I would calm you down in preparation for tonight's show, and tell you that there is absolutely nobody out there tonight in the audience. Just my husband Jack, and I…and the bar man."

"Brilliant! Thank you!" I exclaim as Nichola returns to her seat opposite the bar, arms outstretched to make the venue look busy.

"Oh no!" I quietly mutter to myself, whilst pinning my wig to my head, this is going to be a difficult show with no audience, but…. the show must go on! I somehow manage to wing extra comedy banter, to the three encouraging faces, using this challenge as an opportunity to learn more 'on the spot' comedy improvisational skills. Tonight, also happens to be my birthday, and like a gift from god, the venue slowly begins to fill up to maximum capacity.

This was the best birthday present I could have ever wished for, and the audience ended the night singing "Happy birthday" to me, which the bar man encouraged, as a thank you for building and keeping the crowd entertained.

The biggest fear as a comic is that you might not get paid. Not just because of the quality of your act, but as highlighted, because venues may not have enough audience members in, or indeed for some other political reasons. I was performing a 'Jessie J Tribute' gig in a large holiday camp, and as I stood centre stage, a small eight-year-old blonde-haired child wearing circular rimmed glasses, came to the front of the stage and started brandishing an illuminous lightsabre…at my crotch! He succeeded in his mission and upstaged me, as I sang my opening number 'Price tag'. His parents were nowhere to be seen, in fact no one even thought to remove the child from the stage. Staying in character, I finished the song with, "And a huge thank you to the 'milky bar kid' now could someone come and collect him before he does some serious damage!"

The room belly-laughed at my quip, and I regained control of my show.

However, at the interval the manager of the venue came to see me and said, "You were hilarious, how you kept in character whilst that boy did that to you, but the parents want you to apologise to them for calling their child 'the milky bar kid' and I'm afraid I can't pay you until you do."

The things we have to do for money!

Another gig in Liverpool began with an audience member outside my dressing room saying, "Listen love, you look very posh in that dress, so I thought I'd warn you that you will get lynched in ere, if you don't sing the lyrics, "Are we human…or are we scousers!"

Great advice. The crowd erupted!…And thankfully I got paid!

A most memorable and privileged performance was in June 2012, when I was invited to perform as a 'Jessie J Tribute Act' at a 'street party' for the 'Queen's Jubilee Street Party', in my hometown, on Northway, the very street that I grew up on.

I was more nervous performing in this show than any other, as the audience consisted of all my family members, friends and neighbours from down my own street. We were all anxious about the weather staying dry, and the sound system speakers being able to carry sound well enough outside.

I transformed into the character of 'Jessie J' inside my uncle Gerald's house, across the road from the line of deck chairs, which had now formed along the entire street. As the audience awaited the show in excited anticipation, I felt the enormous pressure inside!

Costumed in character, wearing black leotard and tights, six-inch heels, black bobbed wig, red lipstick and black nail varnish, and now aged thirty-seven, I gulped…as did my Auntie Carole!

With a surge of adrenaline, I strutted outside in character into the middle of the road on my own street. Remembering my childhood near car accident at aged three, I looked left and right before I started singing!

News about the show spread to neighbours from other streets, and they all came and joined in. Even the local fire brigade turned up to watch. With lots of audience participation, it was so exciting to perform and make people laugh on my own childhood street. Laughter really is the most rewarding gift from an audience, and this appreciative crowd were all singing and laughing and heckling, and waving their flags having fun. As always, I barely took a breath throughout the entire show, in fear of making a mistake, and I couldn't stay long to enjoy the party afterwards, as I had to dash off and drive to perform an evening show.

All the show's credit went to Auntie Carole and the other wonderful neighbours on Northway, for organising the event.

I was so grateful to have been given a two-year contract at both The Cliffs Hotel, and The Claremont Hotel in Blackpool. They were absolutely wonderful venues to perform in, and I loved every minute. My opening night performance at The Cliffs Hotel, was to be my audition by the company director, and it would determine whether I would be booked again. I was told by the director that 'the audience will decide', and if they said that I was good enough, then I could stay.

Understandably, my nerves flew to the surface that night, because The Cliffs Hotel audience was predominantly made up of elderly northern ladies, who were very honest, and could be very unforgiving, with their main interest being in playing 'bingo' at the interval.

I was fortunate that my talented friend, Paul Humphreys was comparing and bringing me on stage that night. He calmed my nerves by making me laugh, before opening the curtains, presenting me like a prize in the generation game. The show was going well, and the bingo was a roaring success, and as such the guests stayed for more. At the end of the night, Paul and I closed the show with a 'Take That' number.

"Relight my fire!" Paul sang.

"Well, you've got to be strong enough to walk on through the night!" I enter the stage for the final time tonight through the bright sequinned curtains, singing in my best attempted 'Lulu' voice.

All was going well, until…

"You've got to have soap in your hole!" I belted out loudly.

Paul's look spoke a thousand words, and none of them were in our duet!

And that was it, we connected instantly through corpsing, with tears rolling down our cheeks, whilst managing to maintain enough professionalism to carry on no matter what…and that was indeed a "Carry on!"

I thankfully got away with my spoonerism, and perhaps because of it, I was booked for the next two years! I was once told that I was too 'classy' to perform in certain venues. I now understand that it was meant as a compliment, but I didn't want to be considered 'classy', so I honed my stand-up skills to be able to hold my own within any and all crowds. Army Barracks gigs became a firm favourite, and as a seven-stone woman walking into a room full of drunken army officers, this may seem rather terrifying for some, but for me it was the biggest buzz ever.

"Hey pretty lady come and sit on my lap!" heckles a man at the back of the room. "Sit down! It's past your bedtime, does your mum know you're up at this hour?"

Entering the stage to an uproar of laughter with the crowd onside, is the only way to start a show, and the reason why stand-up comedy is the best job in the world. A huge thank you to the brilliant Stand-up Comedian Frank Skinner, your rapturous applause started my career.

I first met Cathy in 2011 in the entertainment capital of the North, Blackpool. We were both working in a hotel providing entertainment to the hoards of unwashed holiday makers, who would pile into the Caberet lounge every Sunday evening. I was working the sound and lights from the wings and compering, and Cathy arrived nervously to tackle the hard rock face of light entertainment.

And it is hard! This isn't a pub audience that ignores you, or a theatre audience that gives you their full attention and hangs off every word. This is a room full of families. Toddlers to pensioners. Inebriated parents and bored children…a mix from hell!

Cathy was met immediately with my warped sense of humour when I decided to rename her Jean Claude Van Dome. As she has a razor sharp, self-deprecating wit herself, she didn't even flinch at this and I knew we'd get on!

On her first night, just before I introduced her on-stage, I sensed she was a little nervous as she peaked through the curtains at the baying crowd.

"Nervous?" I enquired.

"A little!" she admitted.

"Is your bum going '50p/20p?' I said, using my thumb and forefinger to indicate a twitchy bum hole. She burst out laughing and during this fit of laughter I introduced her on-stage.

This then became a little tradition we had. Each night during my off-stage introduction, I would make the little 50p/20p hand gesture and she would walk on stage laughing!

Sunday nights were always fun, but usually for all the wrong reasons.

Rude parents would talk loudly through the show, as their small children would wander across the stage. Sometimes the children would actually stop mid-way and sit cross-legged at Cathy's feet, as though they thought she was head of the kids' club!

Of course, where other singers may have been thrown by this, Cathy would just involve them in her show. They would be swept up by her enthusiasm and before they knew it, they'd be her backing dancers!

Cathy was always a ball of fun and enthusiasm, and I don't doubt for a second that she will be back on stage again at some point in the near future!

50p/20p! x

Paul Humphreys - Actor: Dodger (CBBC), Power of Parker (BBC), Toxic Town (Netflix), Coronation Street (ITV) and Singer/Entertainer

CHAPTER NINETEEN: My Theatre School and ME
Sparkle! As there's no business, like show business!

"We don't stop playing because we grow old...we grow old because we stop playing." - George Bernard Shaw.

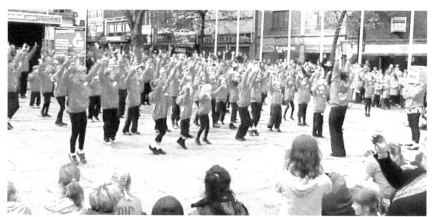

Catherine Vandome with over a hundred of the 'The Sparkle Theatre School' students (age four to twenty years), dancing in the opening ceremony of the '2012 Olympic Torch Event', in Preston Town Centre.

I like to think life affirming moments are hidden somewhere in your memory forever, however indistinct they may seem at the time.

I suppose there's a reason why I can remember being passed a phone, aged twelve, by my mum and being told there was a drama teacher moving to the area, who wanted to speak to me. Little did I know the woman on the end of the phone was to be one of the key figures in my teenage years... That woman was Cathy.

I was a relatively traditional twelve-year-old boy - I liked football, the Simpsons, computer games, and playing out with my pals. I also had a passion for making people laugh. I loved it.

A year before that phone call, I had been in a local amateur dramatic production of 'Peter Pan' as a bungling 'Smee'...I drank it in. I loved being on stage and making people laugh. Nevertheless, as a twelve year-old kid, I did the show and then went back to my normal life. I didn't know how to repeat that process, or feed that passion for drama - until I was passed that phone.

Cathy told me that she was starting a new theatre school in the area and that my name had been passed to her. She told me all about training in theatre, and exams, and developing craft and skills in the arts. It was a world opening up to me. I said I was interested - I really was, and from then on, every Wednesday for five years or so, I spent this time learning, laughing and playing the fool in Cathy's drama school.

It is only now, reflecting on this time in my life, I can quantify what Cathy and her theatre school did for me. I spent my formative teenage years at a sports-mad all-boys school. It was tough, it was masculine, and it was very traditional. It didn't really fit. I liked sports, I was football mad, but I wasn't particularly good at playing them. I liked Maths, I liked Science, but I wasn't brilliant at them either, but I loved Drama. Except that there was no outlet for that. Sports were rewarded heralded, excellent academics too, but not really creativity. There was no drama department, no theatre clubs.

I had my mates at school, and we got on with it. My week was pretty standard, except for a couple of hours on a Wednesday evening. That was when I really fitted in.

Cathy would lead sessions of drama that pushed my creativity skills, and boundaries, whilst also having fun. She would bounce (literally) around the room, bringing us out of our awkward teenage selves. Her energy and enthusiasm were infectious, and it was impossible not to respond.

Most importantly, for the years I went to Cathy's classes, she always encouraged me to be more. I had started because I loved comedy. Cathy also taught me serious acting, she encouraged me to do exams, and to trust my ability and myself. I loved doing my own thing, she encouraged me to lead groups, and do ensemble, and be empathetic. I learned so many life skills in those classes.

I can still recall with huge detail the hours of fun we had in those groups, knowing that Cathy would be holding her stomach laughing on the side of the stage, as I played up to the audience as Puck in 'A Midsummer Night's Dream', or flapping cabaret feather wings in a 'Summer Theatre School'. I performed with a freedom that I have never had in other areas of my life. I sang, I danced, I did drag, I did serious acting, I did anything that was thrown at me. I was great at some of it, and useless at others, but I did it because Cathy had created an environment where I had all the confidence I needed.

By age sixteen, I had already been on stage in numerous roles, under Cathy's tutelage and was (probably insufferably) self-assured. I was more confident, more convinced about who I was and how I didn't need to fit in (in a traditional sense). I could be at an all-boys' school, play football at break, try hard in History or Biology, and 'also' be obsessed with drama. I wasn't quite strutting through the school grounds in the pink dress I wore for a 'Sheila's Wheels' sketch, or the slick back gelled hair I adorned as the evil dentist in 'The Little shop of Horrors', but I was confident in myself.

I challenged my school on their curriculum - why didn't they teach Theatre? Why was it not seen as right for boys to study it? It had kept me going through tough years in that environment. I knew there were others like me, with a passion, with creativity, and it needed an outlet.

We got it, as a theatre department was opened a year later. It wasn't just on stage that I was applying these skills, it was in my 'real world'.

When I got older, Cathy gave me the opportunity to teach younger theatre groups: as usual, Cathy saw something in me that I had not seen in myself. I would spend my evenings after sixth form teaching some of the younger groups.

I fed off Cathy's energy and enthusiasm for theatre, and for inspiring and encouraging young people. It was terrifying, but I knew Cathy had my back, always.

One of the proudest moments of my life was at an end of term show, when a young student in my class took to the stage, last minute, and shone with confidence in a role she hadn't thought herself capable of. Cathy gave me the opportunity to experience that moment, and I am incredibly grateful.

Cathy would always listen and give advice and guidance, we would talk about my subjects, my grades and my future.

Most importantly, everybody had a role, a place, something to contribute in Cathy's eyes.

We were just kids with a passion, and that flame was fanned, never extinguished because we didn't look or sound perfect. For those hours in those classes, we were all stars. That is powerful. It was about community, learning about and supporting each other, and having fun. Not every child needs to escape, not everybody needs (or ever wants) to be on stage in front of an audience, but they need to be supported and encouraged, and that is what Cathy did, week in and week out.

Yes, we put on big productions, but we also raised money for charity, we put on self-devised, and alternative pieces, we sang in hospitals at Christmas and performed and had charity bucket collections in ASDA. We didn't 'need' to do that as part of a theatre school. We could have just done one big show a year, and our parents would come and cheer us on and we'd go home. But there were kids from all different schools, and backgrounds, and talents. It was a genuine community.

I developed a confidence through drama and teaching, that is still invaluable to me. That confidence has been the foundation on which I have built my career and part of my modern self.

At eighteen years old, there was only one thing I wanted to be - an actor. It was my passion. I thought if being an actor was anything like my experience in Cathy's drama school, well I was going to be set for life. I had no idea what to do, or where to go though.

I left Preston and travelled alone to South Africa to teach drama and English. For a traditional kid from Preston, that was life changing. I learnt an immeasurable amount about the world and myself - and I would never have had the skills and confidence to do that without Cathy or the theatre school.

I did go to university, eventually becoming president of the 'Theatre Society' and then the elected president of the Student Union. When I look back on those elections, standing on a stage in front of 500 students fighting for their vote, or pounding the campus pavements, getting attention for the causes I was passionate about, I reflect on the foundation of those drama lessons. How important it is for young people to have a mentor, a teacher, a coach who believes in them.

I was lucky, I had a supportive family and circle of teachers and friends. However, crucially, I had Cathy, and the impact she had on my formative years, if you'll pardon the pun, was nothing short of dramatic.

When I found out Cathy had been diagnosed with ME, and understood more about it, I couldn't understand. My memory of Cathy is somebody who's energy was endless. I would go into those lessons with a glum teenage look on my face, and leave an hour later with a spring in my step.

I know things have been a challenge for Cathy, but it does not surprise me that Cathy has taken her diagnosis as a push for her to do more for others, to challenge stigma and to use her talent to fight for more support and understanding for ME sufferers.

Cathy is unique. The world could do with a lot more people like her.

Sam Butler - Solicitor and proud 'Sparkle Theatre School' alumni and former teacher

After a decade of living in London, I returned home to Preston, like Dick Whittington, but without the cat! I started building connections within the community, and I was very fortunate to be introduced to teaching drama, by my talented actress friend from childhood, Melanie Ash.

Mel recommended that teaching drama was a more stable way of working in this profession, whilst I built up connections in the northwest entertainment industry. Thanks to Mel's advice, this was one of the best decisions of my life. I absolutely loved teaching, and it soon became my whole world.

In 2004, I set up 'The Catherine Vandome Theatre School', later called 'The Sparkle Theatre School' in Preston, Lancashire, and with initially just ten children. My Theatre School was set up on a road called 'Broadway' and with each show, I would tell the students that "Tonight you will be performing on Broadway!" I ran a main Theatre School for the whole community, providing Drama, Singing and Dancing weekly classes for ages 4 - 20 years, as well as running daily 'After School Drama Clubs' in local Primary and Secondary schools. During the holidays, I added a 'Summer Theatre School' and an 'Easter Theatre School.'

Over the next ten years, the business grew and expanded throughout the Northwest, and as a workaholic, I soon filled up any gaps in my calendar with more work. I added 'Half term Theatre Schools' and weekend 'Sparkle Birthday Parties' as well as working for the Lancashire County Council (LCC), and giving 'Guest Theatre Workshops' within the local Primary and Secondary schools' curriculum. The foundation of my 'Theatre School' was to build children's self-confidence and encourage teamwork skills, and it was open to everyone in the community. My Theatre School slogan was 'Every child matters' and they really did. It was an inclusive school and I wanted everyone to be treated equally, and have the same opportunities on the stage, by all taking turns to play leading roles in different productions.

To be less formal in class, local Dance teachers often called themselves Miss 'Forename' and so I decided to call myself 'Crazy Cathy' which derived from a comedy improvisation game using the first letter of your name, followed by a comical description of yourself!

Opening school assemblies with, "Good morning everyone, I'm Crazy Cathy!" with the parroted children's reply "Good morning…Crazy Cathy!" always provided much laughter and excitement from the children and teachers, with only the odd miserable Headteacher muttering under their breath at the informality of it, and tutting with dismay at the 'sudden joy' being brought onto the children's faces. This comical name stuck with me, and the children and parents all called me 'Crazy Cathy'. Indeed, parents would often telephone me outside of school hours, and say "Hello, please can I speak to Crazy Cathy" which always made me smile!

Teaching theatre skills to children, and watching them grow in confidence over the years, was an absolute joy, and I learned so much from them all. Every child mattered, and they all inspired me. I was so proud of them and with much resounding laughter, we were like one big happy family.

Over the years, we staged many genres of theatre including Musical Theatre, Stand-up comedy, Dance shows, Solo and Group singing performances, CD voice audio and singing recordings, live Improvisation (in Asda!), an entire Theatre School (approximately 100 students) flash mob dance routine opening Preston's 'The Olympic torch Event 2012', and two red carpet film productions staring all the students, at the local cinemas.

Every year, I would try to create a brand-new production theme, and invite a wealth of leading Theatre Professionals from all over the world to teach at my 'Summer and Easter Theatre Schools'. I would prepare new ideas for my 'Theatre School' twelve months in advance, to ensure maximum interest for everyone involved, and it was common to spend my one-week summer holiday abroad writing a summer school 'script', whilst choreographing 'dance routines' on a sun lounger in Spain! The professional workshops included; Circus Skills, Stage Fighters, Magicians, Gymnastic Performers, Opera Singers, Puppeteers, Mask makers, Dancers and Choreographers (including Ballroom, Salsa, Latin American, Contemporary, Ballet, Jazz, Tap, Modern, and Street Dance), Rubber Sword Fighting, Film Makers, Directors, T.V. Actors, Radio Presenters, Costumiers, and Special Effects Makeup Artists.

In the ten years of running my school, I was constantly creating and writing new material for the shows, as well as devising and performing in my own evening stage shows. 'The Sparkle Theatre School' was my world.

I was so involved with my 'Sparkle Theatre World' and wanted to ensure that everyone was happy, both students, parents and audiences alike, that I was once jokingly told that I "had little idea of what was happening in the 'real' world, as I lived in a 'Sparkle bubble!' … but I was so proud of that.

I was four years old and desperately wanted to be part of the drama group which Cathy ran at my primary school. At the time you had to be five to join, however, I begged my mum to enquire and Cathy was more than happy to let me join the group.

162

A couple of weeks later she mentioned an 'Easter Theatre School' that she was running called 'The Extra-ordinary Factor'. I asked to come and made it clear that I wanted to play Simon Cowell. Despite the fact that the rest of the group were a bit older, Cathy agreed and made me a 'star.'

The show was a roaring success in the eyes of many and Cathy worked tirelessly, as always, to ensure that it was professional and of a very high standard, which it was!

The feedback was overwhelmingly amazing and I (apparently) stole the show, thanks to the total commitment and belief that Cathy had in me from day one, and it was much more than "distinctly average!"

Thank you,

Isaac Craig - Age sixteen years and 'Sparkle Theatre School' student from 2008 - 2013

"I would go back to this time of our lives in a shot! Loved your shows and your passion, and how much you gave these kids. You should be very proud of giving the best start in drama! You definitely were 'Simply the best!' Wouldn't change a thing. X"

Karen Craig - Sparkle Theatre School Parent, Isaacs Mum

"Party Rockin' in the house tonight... everybody just... shake that!" The loud thumping party music pumps out of the P.A. speakers surrounding Preston's City Centre. It is the '2012 Olympic Torch Event', and my 'Sparkle Theatre School' has been invited to open the outdoor performance, just prior to the Olympic Torch being carried through the Town Centre. A sea of one hundred 'Sparkle Theatre School' red hoodies began dancing my high impact choreographed routine, positioned in rows throughout the Preston cenotaph, directly in front of me, as I mirror their enthusiastic performance.

My heart is in my mouth, and as always, I'm dancing on adrenaline and fear of failure. I don't want to let anybody down. Last night I had no sleep, due to repeatedly jumping out of my bed to practise this vigorous full impact ten-minute dance routine, as though my life depended on it! As the conductor of my own orchestra, I know that if I put a foot wrong today that the entire performance will be ruined. A disappointed theatre school parent, though not as terrifying as a frustrated old lady at The Cliffs Hotel, after accidentally unplugging the bingo machine halfway through 'calling the numbers', was one of my biggest fears.

Rehearsing over the last few months in their individual groups of twenty, this was the first time the entire theatre school aged 4 to 20 years, from throughout Lancashire, had performed this dance routine all together. My teenage flash mob, dressed as integrated members of the audience, enter the stage to a huge 'gasp' as a pram is upturned and a petite teenager inside, dressed as a baby, is tipped out and starts dancing.

My talented friend and Sparkle 'Costumier' Jeanette Worsley brilliantly concluded the dance with a solo dance moment mirroring the group 'LMFAO' whilst donning a cardboard box on her head. As the music concludes and the group takes a uniformed bow, the excited cheers and applause break out and fill the outdoor thrust stage space, as adrenalized children dart in all directions, racing to find their families and be embraced into their proud parental open arms.

The students were all absolutely incredible. They danced the routine seamlessly, working together as one, and I was so proud of them. All the credit goes to them. I looked up, and drew what felt like my first breath in ten minutes.

Moments later, the 'Olympic Torch' was carried through Preston Town Centre. What a privilege to be a part of this event.

Crazy Cathy. The loveliest, happiest, fun and incredibly talented lady I have ever met. Crazy Cathy was my drama teacher for many years at 'The Sparkle Theatre School', and as it says in her nickname, she definitely was crazy and very fun to be around.

She helped me grow in confidence on stage and helped me overcome some very personal issues in my life, that I will always be grateful for.

Cathy always loved every single member of the theatre school, and always put them first.

I thoroughly enjoyed my time at Sparkle and loved taking part in all the shows we did over the years.

My personal favourite was when we did a flash mob in the middle of Preston town centre, where I was crammed into a pram dressed as a baby, until suddenly I jumped out and started dancing with the rest of the school in my baby grow and dummy; the crowd were in hysterics.

I'll always keep memories of Sparkle very close to my heart, and I was so upset when Cathy unfortunately had to close the school due to her illness.

I wish Cathy a very speedy recovery, and hopefully one day Sparkle can reopen, so that more children get to experience the same fun and laughter that I did.
Charlotte Rutlidge - Entertainer and student at 'The Sparkle Theatre School'

The spellbinding magical musical introduction commences, as I am escorted into the Magicians' small black magic box. It is the opening morning of the 'Sparkle Summer Theatre School' week for ages four to nine years. The children are all seated ahead as our audience is watching the show open-mouthed, with pure anticipation and utter excitement, as to what lies in store for them today. Magician and Illusionist Andrew Green mesmerises the audience with his captivating stage presence and exaggerated gesticulation, as he prepares to saw me into tiny pieces, something so many have dreamed of, but so few have been given the opportunity. I bend my hyper mobile body into the pre-choreographed position, inside the tiny darkened surrounds and await the first strike.

"Are you ok?" Andrew whispers into the box under the loud music.

"Yes" I lie from within.

"First sword coming through."

Oh no! I can't remember which way my spine should be for the first sword, was it bent forward or back? I will guess backwards.

The large silver sword appears on the diagonal in front of my chest, and my breath escapes me. The audience cheers excitedly.

"Next sword coming in…ready?"

I can't breathe, and the lack of oxygen in this position has completely wiped my memory.

"Yes" I lie again, not wanting to spoil the show.

The next blade arrives as I am hurriedly adjusting my position, suddenly recalling the correct position of my head for my safety.

Blimey, I nearly lose my eyelashes!

I manage to contort my body as another two swords enter, before I nearly pass out in a combination of sheer fear and a total lack of oxygen.

I must have quietened, and not wanting to cause any harm, Andrew whispers loudly "Are you ok Cathy?"

"Please let me out!" I quietly gasp.

As quick as lightening Andrew pulls out every sword, slightly earlier than planned, but as a part of the show stopping spectacle to an enthralled audience of over fifty children, all applauding loudly and excitedly and eager to participate. Moments later, the small black door flings open, and I am released from the magic box centre stage to take a bow. The excited children cheer and clap with glee, shouting out at how eager they are to become magicians. My career as a magician's assistant was very short lived. Hats off to Debbie McGee, it is so much harder than it looks! What a time to find out that you are claustrophobic!

I first met Cathy when I joined her drama classes in the 2000's, when I was sixteen years old. Even back then it was immediately obvious how kind she was, and how much she cared about helping people, she radiated strength and confidence and it was contagious!

After I left high school, Cathy asked myself and my friend if we would like to help her with her drama summer school for younger children. Every day was full of smiles and laughs, it was one of the best summers we ever had.

Seven years later, I was diagnosed with fibromyalgia, and just as myself and my family were struggling to adjust our new lives, Cathy popped back up into our lives.

I bumped into her on one of my many trips to hospital, and was shocked to see her in a wheelchair. Even though she was exhausted and completely fatigued, she still radiated an inner strength. After we spoke, I came away feeling confident, just like I used to when she was my teacher.

Myself, and my entire family are so grateful for her and everything she has done to stand up and fight for our chronically ill community. There is no-one else I'd rather have representing us.

Whenever I have bad days and the feelings of uselessness start to take over, it's Cathy's example that reminds me to never give up, and that I am not just my diagnosis.

I am continually in awe of her strength of mind and spirit. Thank-you Cathy for continually fighting for us and being a role model not only for myself and my children, but for all of us who struggle with M.E./fibromyalgia.

I can confidently say that you have had such a positive impact on my life, and I wouldn't be who I am today without it.

Thank you for your hard work helping and supporting people all these years.

Jess Knowles - Sparkle Theatre School student, aged 27 years

At the end of my two-week high energy 'Summer Theatre schools', entertaining children with singing, dancing and acting, running on adrenaline and with minimum sleep, I would collapse in a heap on the floor as staff helped me to pack away all the props and costumes. Parents would laugh at my excitable character and incredibly high energy level, saying that "They found it just as entertaining watching me being animated 'out front' dancing and directing the show, as watching the children."

Many said they were not surprised I was so tired, and wished that they could "bottle my high energy level for themselves."

I would outwardly laugh that I was so exhausted, but deep down I was a lot more than tired. I was very sick, dizzy and breathless, and felt as though I couldn't take in a full breath. I had stomach pains and headaches constantly and an increasing swelling and 'burning pain' on the top of my head. It felt as though my head was imploding. I asked my GP what this chronic burning head pain was, and she put it down to stress, from working too hard.

On 16th December, 2004, I had just finished staging my theatre schools first yearly performances of Christmas Pantomimes, which included 'Snow White and the 24 dwarfs' 'Goldilocks and the 10 bears' and 'Cinderella and the 5 ugly sisters', as I didn't want any children to miss out, due to the drama group's ever-increasing intake, the more that local families learned about it. Indeed, our production of 'A Midsummer Night's Dream' the following year, had more fairies inside than any other Shakespeare performance to date. So many, that I had to dream up new fairy names, with a most memorable moment being from a seven-year-old boy, proudly entering the stage with his hands on his hips whilst dressed accordingly, boldly stating "I'm Fairy Liquid." ...and stealing the show!

One night I got into bed, and just as I had in 1996, I suddenly started projectile vomiting. I could not stop being sick, again and again, before I eventually passed out over the bathroom toilet. I didn't rouse, and as I lived alone, I was so grateful that my ex-boyfriend had come to visit me to attend a friend's wedding, for without him to look after me, I don't know what could have happened. Hours later, I awoke inside the Royal Preston Hospital, laying in a bed, and covered in a blue blanket.

"You are alive Cathy!" My ex-boyfriend exclaimed.

The nurse came in to see me, and pulled back the lime green curtain.

"Welcome back!" the nurse expressed with relief. "We thought we had lost you. You were in a coma and we have been trying to bring you round!"

I had no memory of being blue lighted to hospital, or any of the preceding hours to this point. I was sickly, cold, dazed and confused, and as I roused, I was saddened to hear that I had now missed my friend's wedding.

I had numerous blood tests and scans, and just like ten years ago at Queen Mary's Hospital, nobody at RPH could work out what was wrong with me, or why this was happening, and so later that day I was discharged and I returned home. My talented musical theatre friend, Roz Dunning was a wonderful multi-disciplined teacher who worked for a number of years within my theatre school, and most reliably, she came to my aid when I was very sick. Roz would take my children's classes in my absence, and ensure that the show would go on!

Roz Dunning and I were both invited to work at a summer camp in Preston, which was a charity called 'Medicine and Chernobyl' set up by Chris Wilson. The Charity was supported by my kind-hearted friend Dominic Swarbrick, whom I knew from performing with him in 'The Hall Players Theatre Group'. Dominic was the treasurer and fund raiser in support of the children from Chernobyl. This was an opportunity for the children to come over to the UK for a month, and live with families here in supporting their health, whilst enjoying the summer camp activities hosted by day.

Dominic and his lovely wife Lisa hosted a Belarusian girl, Nina, every year for ten years from being age nine, when she first came over to the U.K. thirty years ago. It is wonderful to hear that Nina, who is now in her late thirties, is still in regular contact with the family.

This summer camp became a yearly event, and I was so pleased to have the opportunity to teach the children of all ages, many different activities. I couldn't speak Russian, and I tried a little each day, as the children were all learning English. I decided to use 'physical theatre' without needing any dialogue, and this became our generic language, which included copious amounts of 'thumbs up' from both Roz and I. We incorporated puppetry, masks, mime and group dance routines, all emulating in a group performance, for all the families to enjoy on the Friday evening. The children were all so receptive and generous spirited in their nature, and constantly exclaimed "Spasiba!" to which I replied "Spasiba!" "Thank you!" I said, "You are all stars!"

I first started drama classes with Cathy age seven years old, and I can honestly say she has taught me lessons that I have carried with me my whole life.
Attending her classes as a teenager helped with my self-confidence and a lot of her students, including myself have gained a life-long friend.
Cathy was always extremely energetic, even the kids couldn't keep up with her!
My fondest memory has to be performing on stage and throughout every dance number Cathy would be at the back of the audience dancing along (much more enthusiastically than we were most of the time) making sure we were all in time doing the correct moves.
When Cathy's health started to decline it was very difficult to see the most animated person I've met, struggle so much and not be able to do the things she

loved, but her courage and willingness to change the stigma behind this awful illness is an inspiration to us all.

Fiona Lucas - Dog Groomer for Cathys dog Tinker, and 'Sparkle Theatre School' student, aged 25 years

The cinema doors fling open, and a formally dressed row of 'Sparkle Theatre School' students and their proud parents are all lining the red carpet, smiling broadly in anticipation of tonight's cinema screening, and ready for a professional photograph. This is our cinema production screening staring all of the theatre schools' Northwest students. It is Preston's version of the BAFTA awards. Despite not having to perform tonight, I am unable to relax and enjoy myself, as I am adrenalized worrying if everyone will enjoy the film, and hoping that the movie won't have any technical issues.

The cinema is hosting multiple screenings of the films tonight, due to the number of students involved. Popcorn box in one hand, and a large fizzy drink with a straw in the other, the excited faces of both students and parents watching themselves and their children on the 'big screen' is rewarding.

Unlike a conventional quiet film screening, the excitement and buzz can hardly be contained, as one by one, each person sees themselves up on the screen and points and giggles loudly. As one set of multiple screenings finishes, the next awaiting Sparkle film stars are escorted down the red carpet to the flash light of the photographer, and the second screenings begin. The cinema manager directs his staff to and from each screen, ensuring the evening is professionally run, and making sure that there is enough popcorn for everyone!

The positive response is overwhelming, firstly staring on Broadway, and now up on the movie screen! I was so happy for everyone both front and back of the film making process, it was another very proud moment, with all the credit going to everyone involved, in particular all the talented students.

I have known Cathy since starting 'The Sparkle Theatre School' in Year 4 aged nine years old, alongside my sister Cally.

After experiencing what the after-school sessions were like, it was not long before I got involved in the Summer and Easter Schools that Cathy also ran.

Cathy has always been a funny and kind person, who looks out for everyone, no matter what.

She aimed to make people laugh through the most simple things, like taking the register at the beginning of a Sparkle session.

Cathy also looked out for people, and even got on stage in place of me, because I was scared, as well as standing at the back, doing all the dances and songs so that we knew what to do.

I also have so many memories that even 10-15 years later, still make me giggle and smile to this day. That is what I aim to do in my daily life.

I don't think I could thank Cathy enough for everything she has taught me. Sparkle gave me so much confidence, and I don't think I would be the person I am today without it.

Cathy taught me so many amazing skills, such as improvisation, and perseverance that help me be the teacher I am today. I would still be the shy girl who didn't believe in themselves, if I hadn't had Cathy or Sparkle in my life, and I am so grateful for everything it has allowed me to achieve.

My love for drama and this theatre school continued well into high school until the company closed in 2014. However, the memories that I made with Cathy still continue to this day.

Looking back, there are so many stories that could be told about the laughs and amazing times we had, however that would take a very long time, so here are a few highlights from all those years.

The first recorded film production that I did at Sparkle was not only entertaining, but special, as we got the chance to see it on the big screen during our own red carpet viewing at the cinema. It was a comedy film called 'The Magic Coin' which followed a rich mother and her blind daughter on a cruise. However, it was anything but an ordinary cruise as we adventured into a dream which included riding on a giant inflatable whale (yes you read that correctly!) Fighting pirates, granting three wishes and donating money to 'Galloways Society for the Blind'.

This was one of the funniest to film and the thing that made it so memorable was not only the laughs we had with the group but, also the use of the giant inflatable whale. I do not know of many people who would incorporate a prop like that!

Another memory that I will cherish is dancing in the city of Preston for the 'Olympic Torch Event' in 2012. Sparkle gave me this opportunity that I would never have had, and thanks to the videos that I will never forget.

I even got to play Cathy herself in a couple of stage and film sketches, which brought lots of laughter to both me and the audience.

In 2014, the last show Cathy ever did was called 'Musical Mania 2' in which I played Audrey in a song from 'The little Shop of Horrors'. This was massive, as it was the first singing role that I had played. I do not think that I could have done it without the support from Cathy, as well as the other cast members, but it will go down in history as something which really developed my confidence.

I can honestly say with my hand on my heart, that I do not know what type of person I would be today if I had not joined 'Sparkle' and had the opportunity to not only develop in confidence, but grow as a person.

Lorna Munro - Primary School Teacher and student at The Sparkle Theatre School, aged 21 years

In memory of 'The Sparkle Theatre School' - (2004 - 2014)

CHAPTER TWENTY: ME too!
Self-Reflection...

"A woman is like a tea bag. You can't tell how strong she is until you put her in hot water." - Eleanor Roosevelt.

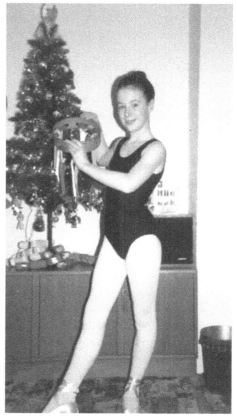

Catherine Vandome aged thirteen, on her Ballet Exam day, at the 'Barbara Saunders Jones Dance School', on Broadway, in Preston, in 1987.

I first met Cathy in 2008, when I worked with her as a teacher at her children's Theatre School. My two children also attended and thoroughly enjoyed coming to the Summer Theatre schools over the years.

I would call Cathy the "Duracell Bunny" because she never kept still. I remember Cathy standing at the back of the hall during every show, frantically dancing and singing and performing all of the show so that the children had someone to copy. It was tiring just watching her!

Cathy's journey is not just about overcoming ME, but she is overcoming all of the toxic situations she has gone through, whilst constantly putting everyone else's needs first.

One time when Cathy had a very challenging situation to deal with, I was simply amazed by the strength of character she had to keep going.

As an entertainer myself, I know that with every fibre of my soul that the show must go on, but Cathy was not letting this stop her, in the same way that she has dealt with ME.

Cathy has always been so strong in dealing with everything, and despite being let down and treated very badly by a number of people, she has never closed her heart off. She is an example to all that ME is not lazy, or a made-up illness, it is a battle to be fought every day, minute by minute!

Even now when Cathy should be focused on her well-being, she is fighting to make the roads easier for those who travel it after her…

Cathy is an inspiration to me and my children and all the children she taught over the years at her 'Sparkle Theatre School' and I would go to the ends of the earth to support my friend, as she has done for me and so many others.

Love you honey x

Roz Dunning - Singer, Compere and 'Sparkle Theatre School' Teacher

Tired and pale faced from my Saturday morning ballet class and cycle ride, I stop briefly on my way home to collect one of my nana's delicious rhubarb pies in a silver baking tray, for my family's dinner. I take this moment to catch my breath. I stand opposite my nana's large bathroom mirror rusting around the edges, and I wince, analysing my vast amount of imperfections.

I am wearing a black leotard and skin-coloured tights, my hair pulled back into a bun with sharp grips pinning it tightly to my scalp, and accentuating my features. I am underweight, but I see a short, fat, white, ugly girl, with rounded shoulders, looking back at me. My joints are so hyper mobile, that when I try and put my knees together my legs bend outwards. I look ridiculous. My stomach is always bloated. I have to consciously hold it in all the time, so I don't look so fat.

I want to change everything about myself. Everything. Apart from my laugh…I like my laugh! My theatrical career is centred around appearance, and as a type 'A' personality, I am over critical of self, and looking in the mirror for flaws has become an obsession. I am thirteen, and I am most obsessed and critical about my appearance during my ballet classes. Ballet dance is understood to be the hardest form of dance, and it incorporates the analysis of one's own body structure; the frame, the alignment, and the mobility, and classes are performed in front of large mirrors to study the entire frame from all angles. I stare ahead at myself in a daze, eyes overflowing. What a shame I have been given this body to live in.

"Cathy!"

I wipe my eyes and bounce downstairs to see my nana.

A hearty laugh out loud in the kitchen with nana, as she hands me her weekly baking, instantly distracts me, and she warns me with a chuckle "Now keep my baking straight in your bicycle basket Cathy, and whatever you do, don't fall off… and damage that rhubarb pie!"

I arrive home and deal with my emotions as I was raised to do, by using humour. I joke with my dad that I have got *his* legs, and he laughs "Well can I have them back please?"

My father, now in his mid-forties, who had in his youth modelled hairstyles for Hairdresser 'Vin Miller', at stage shows at the old Saul Street Baths, in Preston, continues the comedy by telling me "When I look in the mirror, I see a young handsome, slim teenager", and suggests "Perhaps we should swap mirrors!"

We laugh. My mother, in her early forties, wearing a blue and white striped tabard, with a large yellow duster draping from the centre pocket, joins in saying "Eeh! Cathy I have never worried about what I look like, or what anyone thinks of me. Who is bothered about seeing me dressed like this?"

"We are!" My younger brother David comedically pipes in.

With a few jokes back and forth, I am once more distracted and I try to accept my fate.

Three years later, at aged sixteen years, I model with my father on the front cover of a TWS Audio Visual Equipment brochure. TWS was connected to Ingersol Rand (a manufacturing company, who purchased the equipment.) My father modelled up front playing the lecturer using the equipment, and I was sat on the front desk in a mini skirt and heels, studiously holding a notepad and pen, as the so called 'glamorous' assistant.

In spite of this modelling contract, I never once thought that I was attractive, indeed, I believed that I would have to work twice as hard as everyone else in this skin, to be accepted. With low self-esteem, I wore make up every single day, from aged 13 years onwards, including wearing foundation base make up in school hours, as well as full make up and nail varnish in every stage performance.

With long straight brown hair, at that time where '1980's spiral curls' were all the rage, and other children's parents could afford hairdressers' trips, I would sit still for hours on a wooden chair in the kitchen, as my mother (trained by her mother, a qualified hairdresser), would patiently do my 'home perm' herself.

The smell of this highly toxic ammonia filled product being generously applied to my hair and scalp was overwhelming for us both. I would struggle breathing, and my face and scalp would turn red and bleed, but one has to suffer to fit in with trending fashions. I would then attempt to heal my bleeding scalp by generously applying G.P. prescribed Betnovate Scalp Application, and wash my hair in Benzene shampoo products. I continued using these hair products regularly throughout my adult-hood.

At aged fourteen, I was allowed to join my friends and have my ears pierced. I had tiny ear lobes which in 'Chinese medicine' is considered to be a sign of poor health, whilst in 'ear piercing' its known as a 'gamble!' I found post piercing that my ear lobes were very painful and wouldn't stop bleeding. Every pair of earrings I tried, from nickel to silver or gold, caused me pain. I was extremely sensitive to so many things, and I eventually gave up on wearing earrings, and curling my hair altogether. My body image perception was challenged throughout my chosen career in the arts. Indeed, it became a part of my daily routine to scrutinise how I looked in the mirror, particularly before my auditions.

Every morning from 1997 onwards, I would get up at the crack of dawn to join the long line of eager and excitable dancers auditioning for West End shows, all clad in full make up, gracing tall slender physiques, wearing figure hugging leotard and tights, and looking down at me…which wasn't difficult!

This peacock behaviour reminded me of my professional childhood ballet auditions. The dancers would perform ritualistic Demi plies, Battement tendu's and full backbends, to assert authority over the surrounding competition, all warming up by the putrid overflowing dust bins, in the cold winter streets of London's West End. I once again retorted as I had in my childhood, by pinching my leotard out of my bum. I auditioned for anything and everything from TV and films, to musicals and pantomimes, and I was lucky to get through many auditions, but as a perfectionist with an inner critical voice, I always took any rejections personally.

I reflected on my high school days, when two boy's in my G.C.S.E. English class graded all the girls around the table with marks out of ten for 'looks' and for 'personality'. We clearly all took the lesson very seriously that day! I was given a 'six out of ten for looks', and an 'eight out of ten for personality', and I was told that I should be really pleased to have scored the highest rating around the table for 'personality'.

Many years later, one of the boy's profusely apologised for this previous grading, and offered to give me 'one'.

Now at my West End auditions, it was confusing, because one day I was successful at dancing, then unsuccessful at singing, and vice versa, so I couldn't work out the psychology behind this competitive and brutal industry.

I submitted to the realisation that my failure was largely due to my appearance, as well as my own perceived lack of talent, and often this was affirmed by the casting directors, who didn't hold back in telling you exactly *why* you were unsuccessful that day…

"Number 3, Number 27, Number 42 stay behind…and everyone else thank you and please clear the stage quickly…very quickly!"

"Get off my stage and has anyone looked in the mirror recently?"

"At your size, the only part you can play is Jan in Grease…the one that eats a lot!"

"Thank you for a successful dance audition, but after being measured on the wall chart I'm afraid you are too tall for the role" …Yes too tall!

"Your agent has put you forward for the Princess, so would you please stop playing it for laughs!"

"Thank you for playing the drums, the keyboard, and singing, I'm very impressed, but I'm not sure who put you up for this musical, no offence but you're too thin!"

At last I was too thin! I went home elated!

It is now the end of the summer of 2013, and at 38 years old, I am now at an all time low. I am feeling completely overwhelmed and no longer feeling in control of anything. My thoughts are becoming erratic, and I keep crying uncontrollably at everything around me. There is something so terribly wrong happening to me. My memory is fading, and I am physically shaking in a constant state of 'fight or flight'. I feel as though my whole world is crashing down around me.

I am compelled to make the most difficult decision of my life. I arrange an appointment with a private therapist. Compared with doing this, stand-up comedy was easy!

I enter the brightly lit therapy room with trepidation. The room is awash with creamy yellow surrounds, and I feel a sense of peace and safety. I can smell the aroma of incense recently extinguished. The therapist greets me with kindness and sincerity, and in a gentle tone she invites me to take a seat. I sit down opposite her and swallow hard, trying to catch my breath and compose myself.

"Why are you here today?"

Pause.

The enormity of what I am about to reveal is suddenly too much for me.

"Help yourself to a glass of water."

I reach for the iced frosted glass on the adjacent table, and I attempt to sip the cool water provided for such a momentous occasion.

I inhale a shallow breath, wide eyed with fear.

"In your own time." The therapist continues, and settles comfortably opposite me in an armchair, providing me with the necessary space to speak.

My tight constricted chest and head are burning hot. I feel the intense pressure of finally unburdening and telling a professional my deepest secret.

"Take your time."

Pause.

"You promise not to tell anyone." I retort fearfully and guarded.

I desperately want to unburden myself and tell this lady everything, absolutely everything, but I am wound up like a tight spring, and I am terrified of revealing the truth.

"This is between you and I Cathy."

Suddenly, like a damn bursting and a river overflowing, words begin to tumble from my mouth.

"I used to be anorexic." I blurt out suddenly unrestrained. "I had an eating disorder for some time, but now this is something else, I am not hungry, and I can't sleep. I am constantly sick all the time and I don't know why? Things have happened to me that I can't say. I can't say."

"Breathe. Take your time."

Pause.

I inhale and babble jumbled narrative about my life in no logical order, darting around the painful memories kept tightly locked up inside, and blaming myself incessantly for making such a bad choice as to starve myself. All the while searching for the clarity as to why I would do this to myself. Unguarded and unrestrained and lost in my surrounds, I continue to speak at such a fast rate, that I have lost all conscious control about what I am telling the therapist.

Once private words are being set free from my mouth. There is no turning back now. I am being allowed to liberate myself and speak the truth, the whole truth. As soon as I catch my breath, I am suddenly aware of my surrounds. I flush with embarrassment and clench my fists tightly, digging my sharp nails into my palms. The therapist pauses and looks directly at me, deep into my wide eyes, and calmly and nonchalantly replies "You have been assaulted."

"No I haven't" I retort defensively. "I haven't."

I have suddenly lost all control, and I cannot hide from the harsh truth. My heart is beating so fast.

"No, I am here because I used to be anorexic, but now there's something physically wrong with me."

The therapist pauses to watch me fidget left and right in my upright chair, biting my lip and repeatedly crossing and uncrossing my legs and arms defensively, in a final desperate attempt to protect myself from what is at last being released.

"You have been assaulted." She repeats. This time the words don't sting as much, only reaffirm her persistence with her therapeutic quest for the truth.

I look away, staring at the frosted jug of water rippling at the surface, as the balance in the room feels suddenly tilted. It's as though the clear rippling liquid is mirroring my own quivering with fear.

"Tell me about the assaults Cathy."

The therapist has connected my name with the assaults. Not only did it really happen, it really happened to me. I came here to talk about having had an eating disorder, and this therapist has just reached into my soul and ripped out the root cause, which has been so deeply buried inside me for so many years.

No one has ever connected anorexia as being rooted in trauma. Everything in my life suddenly makes sense. I tense my back and shoulders attempting to regain self-control, and I nervously blink back the surfacing tears. I won't cry in front of this therapist. Tears should only be released in the privacy of your own home.

"I can't tell you. I can't tell anyone. It's too much."

The therapist invites me to have a drink of water whilst she excuses herself, momentarily leaving the room. I do as I am told, and sip the water, nervously refilling the short frosted glass, and sitting with the uncomfortable emotions now bubbling up inside me. The therapist returns with a large piece of yellow carded paper and a sharpened leaded pencil.

"Cathy, in your own time, I want you to write down all of the traumas that have happened to you. I want you to write it inside a timeline. You don't have to show it to me. This is for you."

On her instruction, I reach forwards and take the piece of paper and pencil from her, and sit back in the chair attempting to compose my racing thoughts. As I begin to write, I bite my mouth, forcing back the tears which are desperately trying to escape my heavy swollen eyes. The therapist sits still and in silence as I write, holding her gaze respectfully towards the floor. In an attempt not to cry, I look up from the page and force a laugh. "This piece of paper is not big enough to include them all!"

Well accustomed to such predictable defensive reactions, the therapist is unresponsive to my jokes and quietly replies "Take your time, we can always get more paper."

The remainder of the therapy session is in silence, and with each offender's name now clearly written in the timeline on the paper in my hands, I feel a cathartic sense of release that I have never felt before. I can no longer hide from this painful, once secretive, uncomfortable truth.

I believe that I am finally free. The heavy suitcase that I have been carrying around with me all my life is dropped right there in the therapists' room. I look up from my paper.

"I have been assaulted by a number of different people, throughout my life, all outside of my immediate family. I kept this a secret, and no one knows about them. Nobody knows the whole truth. I kept busy every time it happened, and I always blamed myself.

I have also been so sick from being a baby, in fact my nana told me that she once saved my life! I have had years of tonsillitis, and my health worsened during the months after I turned seventeen, in August 1991. It sounds silly, but something changed in my health at this exact time. I remember so clearly that I had really bad flu like symptoms and vertigo. I struggled with breathing issues, heart pain, and choking episodes, and my throat was so inflamed. I couldn't swallow food, it hurt my throat so much, and my glands on my neck were like golf balls. When I did eat, I had bad stomach pains, and I was often sick.

In November 1991, I was diagnosed by my GP with Glandular fever and I had to take eight weeks off college, in bed and housebound. I missed a lot of my studies and my 'A' levels mock exams, which was really difficult. This was the exact time when the disordered eating patterns began, together with extreme cleanliness and OCD rituals, and I became body obsessed. I never like to talk about my first University year at Crewe, because it was the sickest that I have ever felt, with non-stop flu-like symptoms and so many throat infections that I frequently coughed up blood. I had a very low mood and was often tearful, which was so 'out of character for me'. Being so sick ruined my time there. I felt absolutely drained, and I just wanted to come home and get into my own bed and sleep.

At my second University, my cleanliness and perfectionism became so apparent, that my lovely friends there joked that I was 'Monica' from 'Friends!' Every time I am under stress, I cannot eat. I am not choosing not to eat, I cannot physically eat. I cannot sleep, I cannot gain weight, I am freezing cold all the time, and I look so pale and thin. I am eating food, I promise that I eat, I eat McDonalds after my stage shows, so what is wrong with me? My doctor thinks I may be anorexic.

"You may be." The therapist continued "Anorexia nervosa is a common condition which can be used as a means of coping with trauma, and the condition can often be linked to abuse. Anorexia also produces adrenaline, and this

176

addiction to adrenaline has also been linked to patients with this condition. There are of course predisposing medical health conditions, and certain medications which can also lead to anorexia in patients, and in your case you have both, you have been very sick with a significant level of health issues, and you have also suffered a significant level of trauma. You have quite a history of all these issues. I can start by helping you to unpack and cope with your traumas."

Silence.

"Now I want you to take that list home with you, and you don't need to look at it unless you want to, but bring it back next week and with your permission we will start at the very beginning of your timeline. You may not want to talk about certain assaults. You are in charge, and it's all in your hands. I am here to work things through with you."

The therapist finished our session with a gentle mantra, bringing peace and calm into the room and into me, so that I feel in a safe space to leave the session. On my way home, I bite my mouth to quieten the rising emotions, and in doing so, I smile as I recount my late nana saying "Eeh! Cathy! They didn't have anorexia in my day. There wasn't enough food to go around!"

Dear Sir/Madam,

I have been asked to supply a letter confirming and detailing the contact between Miss Catherine Vandome and myself as a member of Lancashire Constabulary, on the understanding that my professional observations of Miss Vandome may prove useful in your deliberations.

I am a lead investigator within Lancashire Constabulary's Public Protection Unit and I head a team of investigators dealing specifically with historic cases of abuse and assault.

I first met Catherine in March 2016, when I had occasion to visit and commence an investigation on her behalf into historic events of concern. Whilst I found her to be a warm and friendly person with a kind and welcoming disposition, I quickly detected that there were underlying issues of health and well-being which had a significant bearing on the evidence-gathering process.

Catherine was invariably enveloped in a blanket and duvet on her lounge sofa and clearly experiencing difficulties with movement or indeed noise. Her attention span seemed limited, and she would become desperately tired after only short periods of time. Her memory and recollection of events was remarkably good, but the effort required in recalling those incidents seemed to sap every ounce of life she had mustered in preparation for my visits.

The product of my visits was always going to be a statement detailing incidents worthy of investigation and whilst a detailed testimony of this type may take a few hours to complete, the obvious difficulties with Catherine delayed the completion of the document by many months.

Cathrine appeared desperately bereft of energy and vigour, which seemed so at odds with the little I knew of her past as a performer, dancer, singer and entertainer. She explained about her medical difficulties and discussed the help she was receiving in the desperate hope of returning to a life full of zest. In fact, this would be a common theme in Catherine's outlook, and even today she seems confident that she might one day be able to achieve this objective. She clearly has no shortage of hope and desire in this respect, and I have always been quite impressed by her sheer determination.

There is however, no avoiding the only too obvious and unavoidable observation that Catherine is very unwell and has been for a long time, her recovery would appear to be slow and beset with setbacks and relapses brought on through no fault of her own. These factors were instrumental in my assessment of Catherine as a victim/witness, and it was with a heavy heart that I felt compelled to conclude that she would not be in a position to withstand the rigours of the criminal justice system and most probably any effort to attempt this would undoubtedly be detrimental to her health.

This is not a step taken lightly especially considering the various levels of help and support available to assist victims/witnesses in the court arena today, but I believe her condition was such that I had no choice but to deny Catherine the opportunity to experience personal justice purely based on her acute/chronic state of physical health.

My only other observation concerns Catherine and her strength of character, unlike many people of my professional acquaintance who are struggling with chronic health issues, Catherine has a burning desire and rock-solid determination to rid herself of this debilitation and resume a full life, but at this time and no doubt for the foreseeable future Catherine will have to accept that she is seriously restricted by her disabilities.

I hope my contribution to your deliberations has proved useful and I remain available to assist further if needs be.

Yours faithfully,

David Groombridge
Lead Investigator Operation Fervent.

CHAPTER TWENTY-ONE: Campaigning for ME
Political support for my ME mission!

"The best politics is right action." - Mahatma Gandhi.

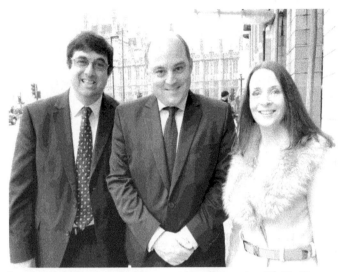

Catherine Vandome at the Houses of Parliament, with Dr Raymond Perrin and The Rt Hon Sir Ben Wallace, Conservative MP for Wyre and Preston North, in October 2017.

I first met Miss Cathy Vandome in June 2017. At that time she was housebound owing to the severity of her ME symptoms. Cathy had previously been a highly active entertainer and stand-up comedian, and she was struggling to come to terms with the debilitating effects of her condition.

I have always been impressed by Cathy's determination to recover. She has been in regular contact with me over the years, and I have assisted her with her campaign to have ME recognised through as a physical and not a psychological condition.

Cathy introduced me to Dr Raymond Perrin who has been instrumental in her recovery process.

Dr Perrin practises 'The Perrin Technique', a manual method which assists the drainage of toxins from the body.

Cathy is keen to see Dr Perrin's treatment included in the NICE guidelines as a recommended treatment for ME, so that other patients can be supported in this way.

I was pleased to meet Dr Raymond Perrin and my constituent, Catherine Vandome, at the House of Commons. Dr Perrin has been studying ME and Chronic Fatigue Syndrome for almost thirty years and has developed a technique for treating the condition.

Cathy is a Patient Advocate who has brought his work to my attention.

A fortnight ago his colleagues published their research on using physical signs to assist in diagnosing ME/CFS. This technique could lead to quicker treatments for patients. I am seeking to facilitate a meeting with the National Institute for Health and Care Excellence to call on them to consider approving the use of this technique by the NHS.

Dr Perrin has advanced the evidential base in this field which potentially offers hope to hundreds of sufferers. His latest research could lead to the condition being diagnosed more quickly and patients receiving faster treatment. I have recently called upon the National Institute for Health and Care Excellence to consider approving Dr Perrin's 'diagnosis' technique by the NHS.

Cathy is an enthusiastic and relentless campaigner, despite her physical limitations. I wish her every success with her recovery and her mission to help others.

The Rt Hon Sir Ben Wallace - Secretary of State for Defence and head of the Ministry of Defence (2019-2023), Conservative MP for Wyre and Preston North (2010-to 2024)

In April 2017, I arranged a meeting in my home, with my MP and Minister for the Secretary of State for Defence; The Right Honourable Sir Ben Wallace.

"Good afternoon your excellency, the Right Honourable...Mr. Wallace...what shall I call you?" I inquired, as I invited Mr. Wallace and his colleague into my home.

"Ben. Call me Ben." Mr. Wallace jovially replied.

Mr Wallace respectfully sat down opposite me on the lounge settee, alongside his colleague, and listened attentively to my case. My little dog Tinker sat on his bed in front of the fire, chairing the meeting. I was waiting for him to bark and declare "Order, Order!"

"I am campaigning through Parliament, because I want to discuss the possibility of updating and changing the current NHS NICE guidelines for ME and fibromyalgia, from a psychological condition to a physical condition, to help save lives." I explained.

"The current NICE guidelines for the treatment of ME, include CBT (Cognitive Behavioural Therapy) and GET (Graded Exercise Therapy) and pharmaceutical medications. I found that all of these exacerbated my symptoms." I continued.

"Cathy, you are the first constituent to contact me and approach me to discuss the condition ME, and I thank you for your emails over the years." Mr Wallace politely replied.

"I am being treated by Neuroscientist and Osteopath Dr Raymond Perrin, who has had over thirty years of scientific research and hands-on treatment of patients with ME and fibromyalgia. He also has a peer reviewed and clinically trialled 'aid to diagnosis' and a peer reviewed treatment for the condition. I ask that these be added into the current NHS NICE guidelines in support of patient care for ME, UK wide. Please would you meet Dr Perrin, and hear about his life saving work. Everyone deserves the chance which I am being given to recover," I pleaded.

"I have shared your emails with other Ministers and MPs, and I shall seek to arrange a time to hold a meeting with Dr Raymond Perrin and yourself in Parliament. I shall be in touch soon." Mr Wallace replied.

"Thank you, Mr Ben,…er Ben" I replied.

The 'Aye's' have it I thought, the 'Aye's' have it.

The 15-minute allocated constituent meeting went by at the fastest time for me, and likely the longest time for Mr. Wallace.

I thanked Mr Wallace for his time in visiting me in my home, and my parting words to him were "If a Neuroscientist and Osteopath has a hands-on manual treatment for ME, which he has been using for over thirty years with great success, then it stands to reason that he understands exactly why ME happens and the actual diagnosis of the condition."

Mr. Wallace smiled and nodded in acknowledgement.

On 31st October 2017, following our initial consultation, Mr. Wallace agreed to hold a meeting with Dr Raymond Perrin and myself in the 'Houses of Parliament' in Westminster, to discuss updating the NHS NICE guidelines and including Dr Perrins 'aid to diagnosis' and treatment for ME.

I was still very severely disabled and, against Dr Perrin's medical advice, I pushed myself to travel by train in wanting to represent ME patients everywhere, and prove unequivocally that this condition is physical.

I was helped by a carer onto the train from my hometown of Preston.

The journey to London Euston was so painful, due to having extreme sound and light sensitives, despite being sat in a quiet carriage. I wore earplugs and held my hands over my ears, my eyes were squinting closed in the painful florescent carriage lights. My head felt as though it was being hit with a brick the entire journey, but it was worth it to try and achieve my mission to help save lives.

Dr Perrin and I were invited into the large Parliament building, welcomed by the kind-hearted Chief of Staff to the Minister, Ms Zoe Dommett, and we proceeded to sit down at a table, as Mr Wallace joined us.

Dr Perrin explained to Mr Wallace about his lifetime's work in helping to treat ME and fibromyalgia, and presented supporting scientific evidence to his work. I supported Dr Perrin by highlighting how 'The Perrin Technique' treatment was helping me to recover from very severe multiple symptoms, which were in stark contrast to who I used to be, when working as a professional entertainer.

Dr Perrin explained to Mr Wallace "Anyone can develop ME, but I have found a commonality in highly energetic careers, including Sports Athletes, Entertainers and Army Veterans. These particular subgroups of ME patients, are amongst the hardest hit. The reason being because these groups of people can physically push themselves to the extreme, putting extra strain onto the spine and neck area, which directly effects the sympathetic nervous system and the lymphatic drainage from the spine," Dr Perrin continued.

As a previous Captain in the Armed Forces, this was of particular interest to Mr Wallace. In the Army, comrades carry heavy backpacks, have multiple chemical exposures and are exposed to extremely high levels of stress, all taxing and overloading the nervous system.

"This is precisely why patients who become as severely affected as Cathy, can become bed bound. They cannot physically walk as they have a compromised drainage system leading to a toxic build up within the brain and body, heavily depleted energy, putting extra strain on their organs, in particular the heart, plus a build-up of lactic acid in the body. This is why I do not approve of graded exercise therapy, until the lymphatic drainage system of the brain and spine are much improved with far less toxicity in the central nervous system. It is also why cognitive behavioural therapy, though valuable in support of some patients with secondary emotional issues, would not help Cathy to walk again. Cathy has pushed herself to the extreme, and she has the will to do, but she needs to rest both her brain and her body in order to recover, not push herself harder," Dr Perrin explained.

Mr Wallace kindly gave Dr Perrin and I double the allocated time, and he was very intrigued by Dr Perrin's insight and knowledge in this field. Used to guest lecturing his work globally, Dr Perrin breezed through his scientific research, and like every patient who has had the good fortune to meet Dr Perrin, it all made perfect sense.

At the end of the meeting, I suddenly crashed, I tried to stand up and my heavy legs wouldn't walk. Mr Wallace kindly offered his arm to help me stand, as Dr Perrin quickly came to my aid. With a drooped head, everything blurred as I was helped out, looking drunk after a cup of peppermint tea. There was no denying the severity of my health condition, and how the high stimuli of our meeting had exacerbated my symptoms.

As always, and to keep my spirits up, I laughed as I embarrassingly dragged my legs out of the front of the building, but Mr Wallace and Dr Perrin both remained professional, and looked genuinely concerned for me.

Outside Parliament, Dr Perrin helped me to sit down for a moment. We were invited to have a photograph together with Mr Wallace, on the front steps of Parliament, and in true entertainer style, I managed to stand up briefly to smile for the camera and tried to 'look normal'.

Mr Wallace respectfully shook hands with us both, and thanked us for our time, as he returned with Ms Dommett back into the 'Houses of Parliament'.

I was helped back to London Euston station, where I received lots of 'tut -ut' looks from onlookers assuming I was drunk. Once I arrived at Preston station, my partner Mark carried me off the train and drove me back home. That day had proven that "ME is not what you do, it's what happens after you do it."

As his constituent, Mr Wallace was very supportive of my personal case of very severe ME, and of Dr Raymond Perrin's scientifically advanced research into the condition. Immediately following our meeting, Mr Wallace contacted the then 'Health Secretary' Jeremy Hunt as well as the Head of NICE, and proposed that Dr Perrin's 'aid to diagnosis' and treatment for ME be added into the NHS NICE guidelines.

Three months later, in January 2018, the NHS NICE panel met with ME scientists, medical professionals, specialists, charities and patients, to announce that they were going to change and update the current NHS NICE guidelines for the diagnosis and treatment of ME, by November 2020.

Over the years preceding our meeting in Parliament, I had regularly contacted Mr Wallace with a mountain of evidence, which proved beyond reasonable doubt that ME was a physical condition. I became an Ambassador for ME, and I campaigned within Parliament and on social media, in support of the whole ME community, to try and help raise awareness and provide support for everyone globally. My once seemingly purposeless bed-bound life, suddenly had a 'purpose' which was essential to my own recovery journey.

I sent copies of my own personal records to Mr. Wallace, as I was being examined and tested throughout the NHS. These included an ENT diagnosis in 2016 of bilateral vestibular hypo function (inner ear damage, linked to hyperacusis and vertigo), a 2016 gas safe report, proving that I had carbon monoxide poisoning from a broken flue pipe in my kitchen, a diagnosis of a tumour in my uterus and a cyst in my kidney and multiple infections. Indisputable evidence that ME and fibromyalgia is a physical condition.

In addition to contacting my own MP in Parliament, I also contacted Ministers, other MP's, Health Secretaries, Royalty (including HRH Prince Charles, now King Charles III), and every single service that I could find, to share evidence that ME was not psychological. These included NICE, NHS England, NHS Northwest, Scientific Research Labs, ME/CFS services, Doctors, Scientists, ME/CFS charities, Blood Clinics, Fire Stations, The Ministry of Justice, and the Police. I was told by a medical professional, that in 2010 ME patients were no longer allowed to give blood, whilst patients with depression or anxiety (or another mental health condition), could still donate. As a regular blood donor myself this concerned me.

I discovered that on 10th March 2010 the Parliamentary under Secretary of State for Health; Ann Keen, said "People with Myalgic Encephalomyelitis (ME) also known as chronic fatigue syndrome (CFS) are not able to donate blood until they have fully recovered." This was in order to protect the safety of the blood supply for patients.

I was also informed by a science laboratory specialist, that they cannot run tests for ME on a patient who is still alive, as it involved tests on the spine, and they consequently directed me to a 'graveyard and burial' service contact, for future use! What I found to be most significant from this discovery, was that the science lab said that ME patient research involved 'tests on the spine'.

This linked directly to my own personal research, which revealed that in the 1900's Sigmund Freud found that patients with ME, (back then diagnosed with 'mad hysteria') all have 'spine irritation' and this also directly linked to Dr Perrins' research into the diagnosis of ME as being a 'structural condition involving both spine and cranium abnormalities' found in every single 'Perrin' diagnosed patient case'.

Still indoors, but not wanting to take all this lying down, on Mr Wallace's recommendation in 2018, I initiated setting up an 'All Party Parliamentary Group for ME': (the APPG for ME). I contacted The Right Honourable MP (SNP) Ms Carol Monaghon, and additionally around thirty other MP's and Ministers cross party, to invite them all to the group, and I proposed that Dr Perrin and myself would be at the helm. Ms Monaghon was very grateful for my invitation for her to chair the new 'APPG' for ME, and I explained that Dr Perrin and I would happily be very much involved in the group in order to help ME patients.

I was disappointed that Ms Monaghon initially emailed me to thank me, but unfortunately declined my offer for her to chair the 'APPG' for ME. However, just one a month later, I was pleased to discover that she had changed her mind, and she did go on to chair the group thereafter, which I believe went on to help support ME patients globally, and I thank her for doing this.

On 24th July 2018 journalist Tim Gavell published my media article in *The Lancashire Evening Post* (L.E.P.) entitled 'Preston woman on an ME mission'. The Right Honourable Sir Ben Wallace and Dr Raymond Perrin, both appeared alongside myself, in the LEP media article, which was about my mission to update the existing NHS NICE guidelines from a psychological to a physical condition, and to include Dr Perrin's 'aid to diagnosis' and 'The Perrin Technique' treatment within the NICE guidelines, to help support ME patients globally.

I was extremely grateful to Sir Ben, Ms Dommett, Dr Perrin, and Tim Gavell for all their involvement in my campaign mission, and indeed to all the ME patients, families, specialists, trustees and campaigners globally, who have been fighting to achieve the successful outcome we all managed to attain on Friday 29th October 2021, where ME was at last recognised as a physical and not a psychological condition.

Peter Barry Consultant clinical advisor for NICE and chair of the guideline committee, said that ME is "A complex, chronic medical condition that can have a significant effect on people's quality of life".

The key major changes to the NHS NICE guidelines are now the following;

The 2021 NICE guideline says "Do not offer people with ME/CFS:
* any therapy based on physical activity or exercise as a cure for ME/CFS.
* generalised physical activity of exercise programmes - this includes programmes developed for healthy people with other illnesses.
* any programme that uses fixed incremental increases in physical activity or exercise, for example graded exercise therapy (GET).
* physical activity or exercise programmes that are based on de conditioning and exercise intolerance theories as perpetuating.

With regards to cognitive behaviour therapy (CBT) the guideline states that "CBT has sometimes been assumed to be a cure for ME/CFS. However, it should only be offered to support people who live with ME/CFS to manage their symptoms, improve their functioning and reduce the distress associated with having a chronic illness."

All professionals should "Recognise that people with ME/CFS may have experienced prejudice and disbelief and could feel stigmatised by people (including family, friends, health and social care professionals, and teachers) who do not understand their illness. Take into account the impact that this may have on a child, young person or adult with ME/CFS; that people with ME/CFS may have lost trust in health and social care services and be hesitant about involving them."

After 100 years of ME being misdiagnosed and mistreated, this proud day in 2021, was one of the biggest medical victories of our time.

Behind every historical victory, are a long line of experts and professionals who helped to make it happen. Alongside Dr Raymond Perrin, Paediatrician Dr Nigel Speight is another one of those incredible professionals, who continues to work tirelessly in support of children with ME.

I first spoke to Cathy in 2018 when she told me about her long history of ME and how much she had been helped by 'The Perrin technique'. She re-approached me in 2022 to tell me she was writing a book about her experience, and asking me to contribute some of my own experience.

I had recently been in touch with Dr Perrin, since he had invited me to speak at the annual conference for practitioners of 'The Perrin technique', and Cathy had seen my talk to this conference. I have to confess I personally don't know much about 'The Perrin technique'. However, I have heard of many adult patients who feel it has helped them and I have been impressed by Dr Perrin's sincerity and commitment on the few cases we have both been involved in.

My experience with paediatric ME:

I became a consultant paediatrician in 1982, never having been taught anything about ME. I dimly remembered some years earlier reading Dr Charles Shepherd's account of his illness. He described severe post-exertional worsening lasting a week, if he took his Golden Retriever for a 100-yard walk. I found his account impressive.

Sometime in the late '80s I was confronted in my clinic by a thirteen year old girl in a wheelchair who announced that she had ME. As with Dr Shepherd's account I found her story of post-exertional worsening very convincing and decided to try to learn more about the condition.

Shortly after this Dr Rosie Woods, a local GP with an interest in ME, invited the late Dr Betty Dowsett to Durham and I attended her lecture. It was an eye-opener for me, and from then on I felt empowered and competent to diagnose and manage the condition. The news that I "believed" in ME got around and cases from all over the northeast found their way to my clinic.

For the next 10-15 years things went smoothly. I was strengthened and supported in my approach by a number of like-minded paediatricians around the country, including Dr Alan Franklin in Chelmsford, Dr David Lewis in Aberystwyth, Dr Rashmin Tamnhe in Leicester and Dr Colin Stern at St

Thomas' Hospital in London. Between us we provided a sort of support network across the country for young people with ME who were having trouble getting diagnosed and supported by their local teams. We also helped to protect innocent families treated with disbelief and subjected to Child Protection proceedings, a very distressing situation for child and family. Sadly, all the above doctors have either died or retired, and I have not found enough allies in the new wave of paediatricians, with the result that I have found myself almost the only paediatrician nationally who can be called in by one of the ME charities in controversial cases. One exception to this rule is Dr David Vickers from Cambridge, who has helped several families around the country, including one well known to Dr Perrin.

One problem is that when I am called in to give an opinion on another paediatrician territory, this can naturally raise antibodies on the part of the latter. In one of the worst cases of this scenario, my intervention helped to protect a severely affected ME sufferer from being removed from her family, the local experts having treated her with disbelief and therefore diagnosed her as a case of 'Fabricated and Induced Illness'.

I have now been involved in over 70 cases of families mistreated in this way, in that they were taken to an actual Child Protection case conference. Although every case has been very distressing for the young people and families concerned, I am glad to say that there has been a reasonably happy ending in c 95% of the cases. However, it has not been a pleasant experience for the parents to have their child placed on the Child Protection register for several years, usually with the label of "Emotional Abuse". What usually happens is that Social Services eventually take the child off the register, and presumably chalk the case up as a success!

The basic problem in most cases has been that the local paediatrician either does not "believe" in ME, or simply fails to recognise that the child has ME, leaving the family unprotected by a diagnosis. This leads to the education system pressurising the family over the non-school attendance.

An example of this happened a couple of years ago in Scotland. The paediatrician had initially diagnosed CFS (Chronic Fatigue Syndrome, a weak euphemism for ME), but for some reason gradually retreated from this diagnosis, ending up with a label "Unexplained Fatigue – no organic cause found". Despite the fact that the boy was bedridden and totally unable to attend school, the lack of protection of a proper diagnosis led to the mother being prosecuted over her son's non-school attendance.

Another situation is where the paediatrician believes in what I call the "Therapeutic Fallacy", by which I mean that they feel that they have some sort of cure for ME. In this scenario the paediatrician prescribes some form of "treatment", usually Graded Exercise Therapy (GET) and Cognitive Behavioural Therapy (GET). The patient gets worse rather than better and the paediatrician blames the family for "undermining" the treatment. A further variation is where the patient is correctly diagnosed with ME but then gets worse. The paediatrician panics, and is scared of having got it wrong and calls in psychiatrists. The latter then naturally make a psychiatric diagnosis, such as "Pervasive refusal Syndrome".

These problems do not only occur in the UK. I have been called to help give evidence in court in both Germany and Norway in similar cases.

Having said that, in most cases it has been possible to protect the innocent families threatened in these ways, there are a small number of true "horror cases" where judges have granted court orders. This has then led to the young person with ME being compulsorily admitted to hospital and subjected to "rehabilitation", usually in the form of exercise regimes from a physiotherapist. Parents who object have their parental rights removed. In every case the young person's condition has worsened, and to this day most of them remain extremely severely affected. It is perhaps not an understatement to say that they have been subjected to "Child Abuse by Professionals", and that this has been both physical and emotional in nature.

One of the most infamous examples of this sort of abuse is that of a twelve-year-old boy from the Isle of Man. (I was not involved but have subsequently met him and his family). He was diagnosed with ME in the Isle of Man, and referred to a London hospital where the diagnosis was confirmed. However, a trainee psychiatrist intervened and contradicted the diagnosis. He stated confidently that all the boy's problems were simply due to his having an overprotective mother. Under his guidance the Manx social services took a court order, confined him to hospital and restricted his parents' access to him. In hospital he was subject to total disbelief in the reality of his symptoms and their severity. The nurses would put him in a wheelchair without a seat belt, race him around the ward and then stop suddenly, on the assumption that he would naturally be able to save himself, thus exposing him as a fraud. When he failed to protect himself and fell onto the floor, instead of opening their mind to the possibility that he was genuinely ill, they simply laughed at his discomfiture. They then went on to subject him to a ghost train, in the hopes that he would protect himself from the various frights that he would meet. Again, he was unable to do so. Finally, they decided to subject him to a variation of the medieval test for witchcraft, in that he was thrown into a hydrotherapy pool, again to prove that he was a fake and would swim to save his life. He nearly drowned and had to be rescued.

The case in which I was involved in Germany was remarkably similar, especially in the way she was placed in a wheelchair and raced around the ward. Fortunately, she was not subjected to a trial of the water treatment.

Currently in the UK the number of families being subjected to the lesser forms of harassment seems to be increasing. This is probably the result of the Royal College of Paediatrics and Child Health (RCPCH) having widened the definition of possible 'Fabricated and Induced Illness' (FII) to include "Perplexing Presentations" and "Medically Unexplained Symptoms". Obviously, the family of a young person with undiagnosed ME is a sitting duck in such a situation.

While the picture I have painted is rather a grim one at present, I am hopeful that the new 2021 NICE Guidelines will help to improve things for the ME community. Most importantly they have stressed that ME is a genuine physical *illness. They have also withdrawn their previous (2007) endorsement of GET and CBT. They have therefore completely discredited the always implausible "Biopsychosocial Hypothesis" (one could almost call it a heresy). This claimed that ME was not a real condition but was simply due to a combination of "abnormal illness beliefs" on the part of the patient, leading to the patient taking to their beds unnecessarily and becoming "Deconditioned". Of course, if this thesis were true, 100% of patients with ME would already have been cured by CBT and GET.*

I should perhaps sound a note of caution about too much optimism. We felt similarly optimistic in 2002 when the Chief Medical Officer in his report stated "ME is a genuine illness and patients should not be accused of malingering". What happened subsequently is that the psychiatric movement behind CBT and GET mounted a major fightback, obtained large amounts of government funding for the PACE trial (of 2011) and somehow managed to propagate the above hypothesis.

Fortunately, NICE have now robustly criticised the PACE trial as "very poor" research, and accepted that GET is not only ineffective but often actually harmful. However, the psychiatric lobby are doing all they can to salvage what they can from the wreckage. Worryingly they are beginning to turn their attention to Long Covid, which in some forms resembles classical ME.

A lot will depend upon on how well the ME community are able to use the report from NICE to argue for more resources for biomedical research into ME, and also better education of the medical profession on the subject.

"I once heard a fascinating observation from someone who cycled from Land's End to John of Groats in aid of an ME charity. The Charity arranged for him to stay with ME families along his route. As he handed the cheque over he said "There's one thing about this condition ME that I don't understand. Does it only affect nice people or can it affect anyone and then makes them nice.

Dr Nigel Speight - MA, MB, B Chir, FRCP, FRCPCH, DCH Paediatrician, Durham

CHAPTER TWENTY-TWO: More than ME
Don't you know that you're Toxic!

"The poison leaves bit by bit, not all at once. Be patient. You are healing." - Yasmin Mogahed.

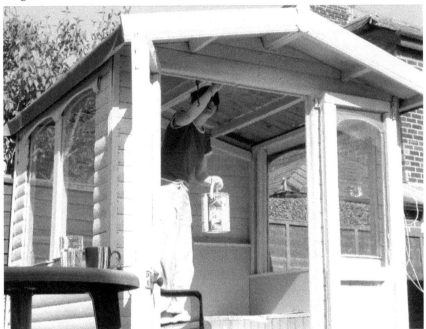

Catherine Vandome painting her garden summerhouse, in June 2012.

What can I say about Cathy that hasn't already been said by all who know her…well actually quite a lot, but it's not printable, so I'm left with this attempt to give you an idea of how remarkable Cathy is in so many ways, in a few words. Cathy, meant in the nicest way, is one of the most toxic patients I have ever seen in over thirty years of running a clinic specialising in chronic fatigue syndrome/ME and fibromyalgia (FMS).

I first met Cathy on 20th May 2016, when she turned up at my clinic complaining of so many severe symptoms on top of the usual physical fatigue and widespread pain, that I immediately thought this patient was going to be a challenge. And boy oh boy…was she!

The toxins had been accumulating in her brain over time from causes such as carbon monoxide poisoning and long-term exposure to paints. Patients who are suffering from exposure to chemical poisons are amongst the worst in the severely affected group of CFS/ME and FMS that I have seen in clinic.

She also suffered from many different viral and bacterial infections since birth, building up pro-inflammatory toxins known as cytokines in her brain, with all the added toxins from the anti-biotic and anti-viral treatments she has had, plus other long-term problems affecting her nervous system such as the vestibular nerve damage in her inner ears.

To add insult to injury, quite literally, she's also had a bunch of allergies and sensitivities including electromagnetic sensitivity (EMS) and Mast Cell Activation Syndrome (MCAS) plus her fair share of emotional trauma, although she did not present with any psychological disorder. There is no question that Cathy has a real tangible physical illness that is not in the psychological/psychiatric camp.

Over the years of treatment I have seen Cathy in extremely disturbing situations as far as her health is concerned, sometimes finding it difficult to walk just a few paces.

We needed to rid Cathy of a life time of poisons. I say 'We' since the treatment is a joint effort…patient and practitioner working symbiotically, and Cathy is a wonderful partner in this voyage we started over nine years ago together.

What has clearly helped Cathy in her journey back to health is that she was very positive from day one. She was clearly physically ill, and with her positivity, grit and determination, she has day after day, week after week, month after month, faced this disease, and is slowly but surely climbing the recovery mountain.

On top of all her heroic efforts, she has been a beacon of light in the nightmare world of thousands of other CFS/ME sufferers and intends to continue her crusade around the world when she is well enough to get back to the stage.

Cathy has become a campaigner extraordinaire in the inner sanctum of parliamentary circles, lobbying many MP's and Cabinet members to take note of her story and my technique.

I wish her well in the future stages of her recovery, and thank her for those many days so full of joy and laughter during the treatment programme.

It has been a pleasure and privilege to know Cathy and an honour to treat such an amazing lady.

Dr Ray Perrin DO PhD - Osteopath and Neuroscientist

Ten years before I collapsed in 2014, I explained to my doctor that I had intense headaches, and that I felt a pressure on the top of my head, which felt like it was burning hot. My GP put it down to stress, knowing the highly intensive career I had, in running two very highly energetic businesses.

In the summer of 2012, after the 'Preston Big Guild Gig', I started to physically collapse off stage, at the end of both my 'Sparkle Theatre School' shows, and my own Cabaret shows. At times I would collapse during my actual stage show, falling off the side of the stage, then I would get back up and pretend it was all a comical part of the show, though I was seriously concerned about why this was happening?

By Christmas, my vertigo and dizziness were worsening on stage, and I had to end my first set quickly and race to the toilets to be sick, without anybody knowing. I came back and carried on, and after a fun show, my legs strangely stopped working and they felt as heavy as lead. I couldn't walk out of the venue, and two strong built inebriated men at the bar, noticed my predicament and offered to carry me. Luckily my kind-hearted friend Jeanette Worsley and her family were all supporting my show, and they helped take care of me, packing away my P.A. system and then taking me home.

I was later diagnosed by my GP with Flu and was bed and housebound, and off work for a number of weeks. Not wanting to let anyone down, I tried to return to work early, and pushed through to teach a dance routine to my Sparkle Theatre School students.

I made light of my situation, and I was laughing with the students that I couldn't walk or raise my arms, but I would be absolutely fine again soon, and I that I would have to teach the classes sitting down for a period of time. The children were all terrific, and in support of me, and we happily choreographed and performed a fun 'hand clapping' dance routine, sitting down on a row of chairs, to mirror my present predicament.

As my physical decline continued, and I could no longer lift my P.A. speakers out of the car, my kind and talented friend Joe Pollard, offered to come on tour with me. We toured the clubs and hotels around the northwest, and Joe helped set up the sound and lights, and before long he became an integral part of the stage show. He would encourage the audience to get up dancing and joining in, and he added extra comedy to my set.

Joe was responsible for encouraging a middle-aged larger set lady, to excitedly copy his professional high kicks on the dance floor, to my singing Beyonce's "On the floor". This poor highly intoxicated lady could not match Joes stamina, and it wasn't long before she ended up backwards "On the floor" the way my song lyrics had suggested!

The best night was after I had performed a two-hour interactive '80s Diva stage show' with everyone in the holiday park up dancing and having fun, I ended the show by taking a bow and pointing to Joe, where he received a bigger round of applause than me…and deservedly so!

During the lead up to Christmas in 2013, now aged 38, I thought 'Mmm, perhaps I'm not using my dominant right arm enough by painting all of my house, holding a microphone, lifting heavy P.A. speakers, and training in high energy sports… why don't I restart table tennis lessons again?'

With a view to entering competitions again, I began table tennis lessons with a private coach. I also simultaneously started with a personal trainer in the local gym, whilst attending regular Zumba classes. The PT workouts were intense. I carried heavy bars on my shoulders and performed squats along the outdoor concrete car park, before returning to the inside of the gym to pull a large heavy rope laden with weights across the floor.

Following this, I would do cardio exercise on the running machine and the exercise bike, finishing with boxing gloves using the punch bag. A tall muscular built gentlemen looked down at all seven stone of me as I was boxing, and joked "I wouldn't like to take you on in a fight!"

I was chasing the burn, and all exercise was starting to hurt more and more over the next few months, whilst my bodily strength was rapidly fading fast.

My PT instructor was getting increasingly worried about me, and he knew something was wrong when I suddenly burst into tears in the middle of the gym because I couldn't do one 'pull up' on the bar and he had to lift me into this position. I couldn't even lift my body off the floor in some sessions. I was completely wiped out.

My emotional state was becoming erratic. I would burst into tears in public places, something I had never allowed myself to do before. I was no longer feeling in control. Sleepless nights filled with terrifying nightmares were becoming increasingly frequent, alongside memory loss, and extreme fatigue. A fatigue that at times caused paralysis. There were occasions when I couldn't move my legs or my arms. It was a very strange feeling. During the day times before I started work on stage, I was painting all thirty of my outdoor garden fences, as well as meticulously painting of all my indoor furniture, coating each piece in black or white gloss paint, as my increasingly fatigued heavy right arm struggled not to shake with the intensity of this project.

As a perfectionist who never liked to ask for help, I painted each item of furniture three times over, to ensure the most professional finish. I had the heating on full blast to help dry the furniture, and as it was a bitterly cold winter, I didn't think to open windows to help ventilate the rooms, and I certainly had no idea there was a broken flue pipe hanging off the kitchen wall!

An elderly neighbour in his mid 90's passed by and saw me up a ladder painting my fence, and said "You will collapse one day if you work this hard! You never stop!"

I wiped my arm across my brow and laughed "Everyone keeps telling me that… but not me, I'm invincible!" I joked.

The following year in 2013/2014 at my 'New Year-s Eve show' in a packed hotel in Southport, I had barely begun my set when I felt very sickly with severe vertigo and breathing issues, and I repeatedly fell on the floor. I was holding my head with a feeling as though I was being electrocuted, and I could hear a high-pitched squeaking sound inside my ears.

I remember this show distinctly, because it was the most physically difficult show I had ever performed with having vertigo, as the audience is constantly rolling towards you in your distorted vision. It was appropriate that I was belting out Tina Turner's Proud Mary "rolling down the river" and I was grateful that my kind-hearted friends Mark Tedin and his mum Gail Tedin, were in the audience, both very concerned for my wellbeing.

I lost my balance so many times, that I joked with the audience that I was wearing brand new high heels and that next year (in the morning), I was going to return them to the shop because I couldn't stand up! I also joked that I was playing musical bumps with myself and that nobody else was joining in!

I didn't want to let the venue down, and so I got back up and carried on the show. I was even given a tip by the lovely manager as a thank you for repeatedly getting back up, and continuing to entertain everyone. At the end of the night, Mark Tedin kindly helped me pack my P.A. speakers away as I lay down in the dressing room.

One month later in February 2014, I collapsed again and this time I couldn't get back up. I was as white as a sheet, under seven stone in weight, and my blood test results showed that I had very low Vitamin D, low iron, low Vitamin B, low calcium, and further hospital investigations showed low cortisol levels.

My GP administered 2000mg Vitamin D, as well as Calcium, Vitamin B and iron tablets. I was initially misdiagnosed by my GP with 'Anxiety' and prescribed Citalopram antidepressants, but these were stopped immediately, due to a severe reaction. My GP explained that "CFS cannot be officially diagnosed until six months after having symptoms, after which patients are put onto a waiting list to see a specialist". I was grateful for being told that it was "all in my mind", because if I'd known I was dying... I'd have died!

Eight months later, I was finally given hope. I went to see an NHS hospital specialist, but he was clearly a stand-up comedian himself, as he diagnosed me with "Likely anxiety". Flopped over a wheelchair dribbling, with my right arm uncontrollably shaking, I begged the specialist to believe me "Please doctor, there's something physically wrong with me, I am not anxious, I worked on stage... I was Jessie J!"

I don't think the last bit helped my plea of sanity, but after some persuasion and my reluctance to leave his clinic, largely because I couldn't physically walk out myself, he then added; "possibly CFS."

Thankfully, a further NHS hospital specialist in the field of CFS/ME, diagnosed me with "Severe CFS/ME and fibromyalgia."and I was consequently given a brain scan in hospital, which I found excruciatingly painful.

I was sent to Pain Management, where together with my GP's existing medications I was prescribed; morphine patches and morphine drink, diazepam, opioids, co-codamol, round the clock paracetamol and ibuphophen (eight of each per day), as well as Mefenamic Acid (for period pain), Fluconazole, Ovex, and additional antibiotics whenever an infection flared. After a year and a half of taking these medications, I decided to stop taking all of them. My GP wrote a letter to the hospital:

"Miss Catherine Vandome has; "Severe incapacitating symptoms. Needs second opinion and advice regarding treating her CFS. Unable to tolerate medications."
GP to Catherine Vandome (2015)

I was told by a number of specialists that I would likely never walk again. One professional told me to go home, accept my situation, and live out the rest of my life in bed. Another said that my career on stage was over. I also had additional tests performed in 2016, outside of the NHS, and these confirmed that I had a 2/3 level of inflammation markers inside my gut.

Over the proceeding years, thanks to Dr Perrin's invaluable support, I was investigated within hospital for additional co-morbidities, which were likely preventing my recovery. Dr Perrin was right when he diagnosed me with ME and fibromyalgia (Plus) other co-morbidities, and this explained why my recovery journey was taking much longer than average. Although Dr Perrins' treatment is specifically for ME and fibromyalgia, over time I found that all my additional 'co-morbidities' were also reducing in their severity.

I was diagnosed in hospital with ME, fibromyalgia (FMS), hyper mobile Ethlers Danlos Syndrome (hEDS), Bilateral Vestibular hypo function, a 4cm submucosal benign tumour on the left side in my uterus (which suddenly doubled in size in 2020, within six months of having two scans), a 2cm cyst in my left kidney (which disappeared on a subsequent scan, after using Dr Perrins lymphatic drainage treatment), high levels of ear, nose and throat infections (ENT), viruses and bacteria infections and frequent heavy periods, with likely endometriosis.

I also had additional health issues from Carbon Monoxide Poisoning, Lead Paint Poisoning, Lead Water Pipes and Damp exposure, Electro Magnetic Sensitivity (EMS), Multiple Chemical Sensitivity (MCS), Mast Cell Activation Syndrome (MCAS), POTS, three infected teeth, internal blood clots, gallbladder, liver and kidney issues, and a parasitic infection. In layman's terms, my stomach was like the inside of 'Mary Poppins' handbag, and I was expecting a lampshade to be drained out next!

In 2016, I had my heart tested in a local gym. I could barely walk or climb the stairs to get to the room for the test. My heartbeat from attempting to walk up the stairs was over 150bpm. Lying down still, wearing a heart monitor, my VO2 max was recorded as 'Elite'. I was astounded to discover that as long as I didn't move, my cardiorespiratory response and level of fitness endurance was the level of an Olympic athlete, and that I have an 'Elite' level heart. Indeed, I believe that this is the reason why I am still alive today. My loving nana always told me that I "have got a good heart!"

My kind-hearted friend, Dave Brand, invited me to his local stroke support group called 'Different Strokes', to see if this may be supportive to my needs. Used to performing on stage in the 'Hall Players Theatre Group' together, we were both now overcoming disabilities, whilst retaining our good humour and cracking jokes at ourselves. Dave said laughingly "Half of my side isn't working, and half of your side isn't working, so if we combine the two better halves, we will get a fully functioning person!"

The helpful specialist running the stroke group noticed that my balance was off, and that I had an intolerance to sound. She suggested that I may have some kind of vestibular issues, and recommended that I see an ENT specialist in hospital. Thanks to Dave Brand, a major issue in my health was flagged, and consequently diagnosed.

Dr Perrin included additional treatments, as well as the standard 'Perrin Technique' due to the level of toxicity I had in my system. In treatment sessions he massaged my legs, arms, and stomach, to get the drainage working more efficiently throughout my whole body, and he would occasionally gave me a 'liver shake' which is like a 'milk shake', but without the dairy!

Joking aside, the liver shake helps to detoxify the liver, and it was extremely supportive to my overall health. Following having 'The Perrin Technique' treatments, combined with a healthy diet, the level of inflammation in my gut improved dramatically.

Over time, Dr Perrin's osteopathic treatment realigned my jaw, neck, back and pelvis and restored the numerous subluxations I frequently presented with in clinic, due to having secondary hypermobile Ethlers-Danlos Syndrome. These treatments included restoring subluxations in my upper right rib cage, neck, right shoulder, spine and pelvis. Twice my pelvis misaligned, and I limped into clinic in pain, and walked out upright thanks to this osteopathic treatment.

I was intrigued to have learned from Dr Perrin, that although the lymphatic drainage system runs throughout the body, it drains towards the left side. This was enlightening as my tumour, the cyst in my kidney, and three of my infected teeth were all on my left side. In 2016, my dentist successfully removed three infected teeth, and years later I had four amalgam fillings removed. My dentist commented that my jaw bite position on a recent scan, was now correctly aligned. He was very surprised to hear that Dr Perrin had manually realigned my jaw using osteopathy.

The jaw realignment stopped my Temporomandibular disorder, (my jaw stopped wobbling), and I no longer had bruxism (the grinding of my teeth), or biting of my tongue and inside of my cheeks when I slept, so I could now throw away my very attractive mouth guard. The jaw realignment also helped to reduce my inner ear pain and my vertigo symptoms.

For my dental treatments, I was recommended to request 'non adrenaline' injections, instead of 'adrenaline'. However, my sensitivities to chemicals were so extreme, that I would collapse after my dental treatments, unable to walk or speak properly.

"Cathy Vandome has been attending our dental practice since 2015.
I recall in particular her last visit to the practice in May 2021 She entered the surgery cheerful and feeling optimistic about her treatment.
Roughly 15 minutes had passed after her dental injection, and I noticed Cathy waving her hand in front of her nose as we were now using a strong-smelling solvent that bonds a filling to the tooth, she then started having trouble breathing and I had to sit her up to catch her breath. It took 5 minutes for Cathy to regulate her breathing. A short time after we were able to complete the treatment.
As Cathy stood up, she became very disoriented and was slurring her words, she needed to be escorted with help from the surgery and wait for her partner to pick her up. She was clearly not fit to drive."
Claire Higham - Dental Nurse Witness Statement - Dental Clinic

Thanks to Dr Perrins invaluable medical support over the years of having weekly treatments with him, he was able to flag several additional medical issues which he requested needed to be investigated further through my GP. I had a major bleed after one particular treatment, and the chronic level of lower abdominal pain symptoms reduced significantly, as the congested drainage inside unblocked. This led to multiple investigations within Royal Preston Hospital and further additional diagnosis' highlighting my health condition to be unequivocally physical and not psychological.

27th July 2018

I confirm from my knowledge of the patient and on review of her medical notes that she suffers from severe chronic fatigue syndrome and fibromyalgia. She is having weekly treatment under the care of a medical provider with a specialist interest in chronic fatigue syndrome.

She has been extensively investigated by a number of different medical specialists and there are no oral medical treatments that can be offered to her.

Indeed the CBT type options again are not something that would be beneficial to her. She manages her condition to the best of her ability by limiting her activity when she is particularly more symptomatic. On most days she is particularly limited in what she is able to do, including activities of daily living and self care. In addition to her condition, she has bilateral vestibular hypo function and this causes problems with her balance, mobility, hearing and vision in particular when she's in areas of high stimulus, such as public places.

General practitioner to Catherine Vandome

28th July 2018

It was a pleasure to meet you in the Preston Genetics on 28th July 2021. We arranged the appointment to consider a diagnosis of hypermobile Ethlers-Danlos Syndrome (hEDS) for you.

You told me that you have had problems since being a small child. As an infant you had a choking episode and you had recurrent bouts of infections throughout your early life. You were diagnosed by Professor White with ME some years ago. More recently you have seen an Osteopath Raymond Perrin who has been treating you with great success. Dr Perrin is concerned that you may have an underlying connective tissue disorder contributing to your problems.

We have discussed that Ethlers Danlos Syndrome is an 'umbrella' name given to many different connective tissue disorders. These different forms of EDS are caused by discreet genes although they often have overlapping phenotypes.

We discussed the most common type of Ethlers Danlers Syndrome is hyper-mobile EDS (hEDS). I explained that the precise molecular cause of hEDS remains elusive.

I was able to assess your Beighton score and you have a significant degree of hypermobilty. You also have a history of painful periods, irritable bowel syndrome and you have had a rib subluxation.

I explained that you would fulfil the criteria for hEDS. I gave you a scientific paper detailing the diagnosis and clinical course of hEDS.

Consultant Clinical Geneticist to Catherine Vandome. (2020 and 2021)

In 2019, Dr Perrins' cranial osteopathy treatments managed to successfully get the fluid moving much better inside my skull.

"It feels like someone has turned a shower on inside my head." I gleefully expressed.

"Only the most severe ME patients can feel this Cathy." Dr Perrin replied. By late 2019, I was feeling improvements under Dr Perrin's treatments, and although my personal circumstances had not changed, my health surprisingly deteriorated in 2020, when I had a sudden burst of flu-like symptoms, breathing issues, heart palpitations, tinnitus, and a worsening of my Electro Magnetic Sensitivity (EMS) symptoms.

From this period of time, I can only describe that it felt like I was a 'battery on charge' being electrocuted all the time, and even more concerning was that I was also spitting blood. I couldn't breathe properly, and I turned yellow, with increased liver pain. I looked like Marge Simpson but without the pearl necklace! However, most interestingly, was that when I went into the woods, the EMS and tinnitus stopped, and I felt at peace. I realised that I was going to have to find a job working inside the woods, although I'm not sure if Little Red Riding Hood gets paid?

In January 2022, a literal 'break through' came as Dr Perrin used osteopathy to pop the C1 in my neck back into place, after which I felt fluid draining down the back of my neck. Two weeks later, he turned me onto my side and popped the L4 and L5 at the base of my spine, at which I let out an almighty scream, followed by tears of joy, as the chronic kidney, bladder and back pain I had lived with for years reduced, and I felt a sensation of fluid draining down the base of my spine.

Over time, I noticed that the structural alignment of my entire frame had changed dramatically. I am now naturally walking taller, my neck alignment is stronger, and my ankle and knee joints are no longer hyper extending. I can now walk comfortably flat footed, (no longer more comfortable in high heels) and I can stand with my knees touching together. My hEDS symptoms were simultaneously repairing. The extreme level of joint hyper mobility has reduced, with far fewer subluxations, alongside a reduction, and a complete eradication in many of the extreme symptoms I had initially presented with.

After a lifetime of non-stop sickness, I am no longer having flu-like symptoms of any kind, no hay fever, or asthma, or gastric reflux, in fact I no longer even present with 'a common cold'. Thanks to 'The Perrin Technique' treatment, the fluid drainage is now flowing much more efficiently, towards the correct direction of flow, throughout my entire system.

Most notably, after decades of recurrent tonsillitis, my neck is no longer inflamed, the 'golf ball' sized glands are gone, and I am overjoyed to say that I have never had this painful health condition since! It really is 'nothing short of a miracle', and with a newfound sense of self-worth, I am no longer describing myself as 'nothing short!'

"Thank you Dr Perrin!" I exclaimed "You're a genius!"

Ever the humble gentleman, he laughingly replied "No Cathy…I'm just an Osteopath!"

On Sunday 28th January 2024, I suddenly fell to the lounge floor crying out and holding my head in pain. It felt like there was something sharp inside my head. I flushed extremely hot and cold, reminiscent of the high temperature fevers which I had experienced in childhood. My partner Mark Singleton looked after me, wrapping me in multiple blankets, as I lay down shivering, unable to get warm. I fell fast asleep mid-day and 'out of character' I slept right through until the following morning. On waking, I felt as though a pressure in the right side of my skull had gone, as though something major had cleared out of my head.

For the first time in ten years, I felt as though I was finally coming alive again. I was no longer deathly white, and people commented that I now had a 'natural colour' to my cheeks, without wearing any make up. I saw Dr Perrin the following day for treatment, and he was so pleased to hear this news.

"Cathy, this is wonderful news, but as you have been so severely affected, I recommend that you 'er on caution' and continue to rest and stay away from anything that could set you back, in order to have the best chance to completely recover and most importantly remain well."

A few months later, I was researching 'magnets' and the possible link to my Electro Magnetic Sensitivity (EMS) symptoms, which were causing me to shake and collapse in high levels of electricity, such as watching a show in the local theatre. I had long suspected that I may be magnetic, and I did a magnet test at home and found that the magnet was sticking to certain parts of my body. I shared this information with Dr Perrin, in Clinic on Monday 15th July 2024. On my request, Dr Perrin proceeded to test my body with a neodymium disc magnet, and was shocked to discover that a magnet was indeed sticking to various parts of my body, most notably on my arms and along my spine.

"What if other ME patients are also magnetic like myself?" I asked.

"Wow Cathy. I cannot believe what I am seeing!" Dr Perrin exclaimed.

"I always knew I was a bright spark!"

We both laughed.

Following my discovery, Dr Perrin said that he would now do further research into this magnetic connection and see if other ME patients were also experiencing this phenomenon.

"Dr Perrin, if you had known that you'd have to put up with me and my jokes for nine years, you may have reconsidered my initial diagnosis!" Dr Perrin laughed, as he looked over to my partner Mark in sympathy.

"Remember that the earlier the diagnosis and treatment begins, the better the ME patients' prognosis. You may need 'top up' treatments for life Cathy, with having had such a high level of chemical exposure, over a long period of time. This will ensure that your lymphatic system continues to work more efficiently, and it will hopefully help to prevent a relapse."

I slowly sat upright on the massage bed, as Dr Perrin wrote up my medical notes for the week. I smiled over at him with gratitude. "There were two men that walked the earth laying their hands on the sick and healing them. One was Jesus, and the other was Dr Perrin."

Dr Perrin laughed. "Don't include this joke in your book!"

So I did.

I first met Catherine or Cathy as she prefers to be known on 23rd August 2017, since that time she has visited the clinic for a colon hydrotherapy treatment for a further four treatments.

Colon Hydrotherapy is a modern and efficient technique used to provide a comfortable and harmless solution to an age-old problem of eliminating toxins. The treatment involves administering warm filtered water into the colon, which promotes the elimination of multiple stored toxins out of the body.

In recent years there has been a renewed interest in natural therapies including colon hydrotherapy. Colonic therapy assists the body's own mechanisms by stimulating the nerves in the colon and helping to improve the motility of the lower bowel, which promotes the removal of stored toxins.

I trained as nurse in 1989, and worked for the NHS and in Private hospitals for several years, prior to opening Wellsprings Holistic clinic, this was as a direct response to witnessing the effects that colon hydrotherapy had on my teenage daughter's eczema.

I trained with an eminent American Doctor and naturopath who promoted the virtues of cleansing and healthy lifestyles, which involved colon hydrotherapy. I now also train others to become colon hydrotherapists, along with running Wellspring's Holistic Clinic.

Over the last twenty plus years I have seen many individuals benefit by colon hydrotherapy. Clients present with an array of different conditions and symptoms such as bloating, bowel irregularity, yeast infections, irritable bowel syndrome, back pain, digestive problems, migraines, fibromyalgia, multiple sclerosis, and myalgia encephalomyelitis/chronic fatigue syndrome.

My involvement with Cathy began in 2017, when she received three treatments in short succession, as recommended by Dr Perrin.

On the initial treatment it was obvious from both her medical history and her appearance that she was not in a good place in relation to her health.

Regarding her lifestyle and eating habits there were no red flags that would alert me to any under lying issues that were not related to her ME.

I was both impressed by Cathy's awareness of her own body's needs and her depth of knowledge attaining to ME. Along with her positive attitude and determination to get well and help other sufferers of ME.

Her digestive system was not functioning efficiently resulting in IBS. She had been to see Dr Perrin who was supportive of her receiving further treatments in conjunction with the Perrin lymph drainage massage.

Cathy returned a few years later for another couple of treatments with me, and I learnt that she had continued to battle with the symptoms of ME, but felt that she was now progressing in her recovery following the Perrin protocol and the regular lymphatic drainage massage that she had received. I immediately noticed that Cathy looked less drained, and appeared quite upbeat about the progress that she had made.

Cathy had stopped taking lots of supplements, and continued eating healthy nutritional foods, but was now eating meals completely prepared from scratch, with no processed foods, gluten, dairy or sugar.

Cathy intends to return for future treatments, as she has found these beneficial to her recovery.

Cathy has made a remarkable contribution to the understanding of ME from a personal perspective. I have appreciated the knowledge she has shared with me in relation to both the physical and emotional aspects of ME, which I feel allows me to have a better understanding of the challenges involved.

In conclusion, I wish her continued improved health allowing her to return to her career as an entertainer, whilst continuing to reach out to other ME sufferers.

Lynne P McDougall - BSc (HONS) Cert Ed. RCT. - Wellsprings Holistic Clinic
www.colonic-irrigation.uk.com

CHAPTER TWENTY-THREE: How I recovered from ME
Heal from Within my fellow 'Magnanimous Empaths!'

"It ain't what you do it's the way that you do it. And that's what gets results." - 'The Fun Boy Three with Bananarama' - UK Pop Group (1982).

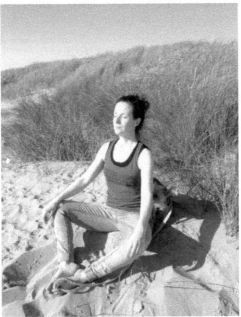

Catherine Vandome practising Meditation on the local beach, in recovery from ME.

I first met Cathy 35 years ago! We were both child performers and although we trained at different dance schools, we knew each other through the various shows we both took part in across Preston and Lancashire.

As little ones we would have been cute little animals in the woods for Panto's and as we got older, we took roles singing and acting - as well as dancing in various Youth Theatre and professional Pantomimes.

At college we met again, whilst we both studied theatre and then again briefly at University.

During our childhood Cathy was always the 'life and soul', she had confidence I only dreamed of and what a talent!

Years later, our paths crossed again when we were both working professionally - me as an actor on T.V. and Cathy as a stand-up comedian and singer.

We found ourselves back in Preston, where it all started, and I introduced her to the joy of teaching - a great way for many performers to support their income.

As predicted, she excelled at teaching and mentoring the next generation of stars as well - and parents and pupils loved her infectious enthusiasm, high standards, creativity and imagination.

Cathy is truly an inspiration - without the health problems she has endured - I would write this in support of her, but knowing some of what she has been through as a human, aside from her performing, I can't help but continue to marvel and hold her in great regard and esteem.

One day I would love to see Cathy on stage again - teaching again and bringing her charm and joy to people's lives, but until then, I am thrilled she is turning what has been a horrendous and traumatic experience into a way of helping others.

Typical Cathy - break a leg sweetheart, love you x
Melanie Ash - Actor and Drama Practitioner

I lovingly recall my nana saying in times of sickness "This too shall pass" … my nana didn't have ME! Recovering from an illness that does not exist, and has no cure, was going to be the hardest job in the world. However difficult the journey was to be, nothing would be as terrifying as living forever, in the level of 'inhumane torture' I was enduring in 2014.

I knew that when I recovered, my first return stand-up comedy show was going to be inside the hospital, because every time I was wheeled into any department and said "I have got ME" I was guaranteed to get a laugh!

I want the reader to know that I am not a medical professional, and I do not work for Dr Raymond Perrin, or any of the product manufacturers which I recommend have helped me. I am a lay person telling my own truthful story, and I am an independent advocate of 'The Perrin Technique' treatment for ME. I spent a lot of money on 'experimental' treatments and tests, before I found the right treatments that worked for me. What worked for me may not work for everyone, but I hope that in sharing my own story and healing modalities, that the reader may have access to numerous supportive tools, that may aid and improve their health also.

I discovered that "Most people don't want to give up today, for a tomorrow that may never be." … I wasn't most people. My recovery journey was like riding a giant rollercoaster. There were extreme highs and disappointing lows, with numerous spinning loops in between. I strapped myself in tight, and I prepared myself for any challenges that lay ahead. My mindset was unbreakable. I was not going to give up fighting to recover, no matter what.

Like riding a giant rollercoaster, I laughed, I cried, and I vomited my way back to better health. There were perks to being disabled. People who saw me sitting in a wheelchair said, "I'm so sorry, I have just used your toilet." I discovered that I was now the proud owner of all the disabled toilets in the northwest!

My recovery journey from ME (Plus other co-morbidities) utilised all four healing modalities, involving the structural, chemical, physical and emotional pathways. I have made a list of all the recovery tools, which I found to be the most supportive on my own healing journey, and I have put them in my chronological order of preference. I hope that these tools are helpful to you the reader, and as every single ME patient is unique, some or all of the following supportive healing modalities may apply and be helpful to you personally.

I realised that I had to make significant changes to my life, because in order to have the best chances to recover from any chronic illness, if we "keep doing what we are doing, we will keep getting more of the same." I learned that the key to healing, is finding the 'balance' in all things. My life was massively out of balance.

I began by manual detoxification, using 'The Perrin Technique' as well as balancing the gut microbiome, by eating a healthy diet. I also incorporated balancing the meridian 'awake and sleep' cycle and the 'work and play' cycle with sufficient rest and sleep, the 'fight or flight' emotional interaction cycle by releasing traumas, the 'boom or bust cycle' with gentle exercise and relaxation, the 'time doing' with others and 'time alone' cycle in setting healthy boundaries, and most importantly balancing the stimulation of the sympathetic nervous system, by 'engaging the para-sympathetic nervous system' needed to rest, digest and recover, through meditation.

The most difficult part of this experience for myself, was not being believed to be physically sick. Therefore, most importantly if you have ME, and you do not feel believed, I want you to know that I believe you and I believe in you. You matter most and you can do this. Recovery from anything is a constant, it is all about consistency in making small incremental changes to our lifestyle choices ahead, in support of attaining better, and indeed optimal health.

There are no certainties in life, but to have the chance to feel better than I did, meant that it was undoubtedly worth trying. We may manage to recover from ME, but we may also have additional co-morbidities or secondary issues caused by having had undiagnosed ME for a long time, which may prevent complete recovery. However, if we set ourselves on the right path ahead, find the right balance in all things, and always listen to our gut, I believe that we all have the very best chance to 'heal from within'.

From where we are today, we are free to let go of the past and begin to enjoy a new life filled with undiscovered opportunities, within the limitations of our present state, and with continued healing ahead... who knows what may become possible? In order to heal from anything, I recommend that we focus on our own journey, and do not be distracted by others. Always remember my life's motto: "Everyone is trying to do their best with the tools they have been given. It's just that some people have been given an excavator!"

To my fellow ME friends, you are truly...MAGNANIMOUS EMPATHS!

1. THE PERRIN TECHNIQUE TREATMENT FOR ME:
In 2010, Dr Perrins treatment was nominated by ME patients, as the third most helpful intervention following 1) Rest and 2) Pacing for ME patients, by the ME Association Charity, who's medical advisor was Dr Charles Shephard.

I contacted 'The Perrin Clinic' for an initial consultation and a diagnosis from a qualified Perrin Practitioner, and in my case this was with Dr Raymond Perrin, and I started my weekly treatments with him. I continued to have these over the following years, as well as his recommended daily self-massage treatments at home. (For further information, please see end of Chapter 5). I found 'The Perrin Technique' treatment to be 'central' to my recovery journey.

2. DIET FOR ME:

Disease: - "Diet causes it and diet cures it" - Joseph Goldberger - American physician and epidemiologist in the US Public Health Service and advocate for social recognition of the links between poverty and disease. (1874-1929).

My diet had always been the least important focus in my life, and now in order to recover, I chose to make it the most. My entire life had been so fast paced, that "I didn't have time" to routinely sit down, eat a proper meal and actually enjoy it. I found the process of eating was a huge imposition to my busy, stressful daily schedule, and I often suffered from acute abdominal pains afterwards. As such, I reached for the easiest and quickest processed and sugar filled food options, to get me through the day.

I was very body conscious working on stage for a living, and particularly working as a professional dancer, but I believe that it was a 'dysregulation of my autonomic nervous system' which suppressed my appetite and led to anorexia, as I didn't actually feel hunger. Indeed, under very high stress levels I found that 'I couldn't eat, not wouldn't eat'.

Initially, the only thing I could focus on was surviving, in being bed bound with ME. I had no strength or energy to physically lift a spoon to my mouth, and I was having severe allergic reactions to any and all foods. Thanks to the support from my carers, they prepared and cooked the food for me.

I had to start from the very beginning, and learn to enjoy the process of eating healthy foods and drinks, from the initial whole-food preparation and the joy of cooking, to the ultimate satisfaction and pleasure of eating and tasting 'real foods'. I was so rehearsed at the Western quick fix of 'reaching for a tablet' be it medicinal or herbal, to reduce my pain or supply vitamins and minerals, that the very idea that many essential cell repairing and immune boosting healing medicines could actually be consumed through optimum healthy diet choices, at first to me seemed impossible.

Over the years, I decided to make cooking a creative process, like making a piece of art to consume. With carer support, I took photographs of the steps of preparation, and posted the recipes and photographs on social media, and this was one of the best decisions I made during my recovery.

Few people knew just how physically time consuming and difficult it was for me to prepare food and eat it, with such limited brain function and depleted energy levels, but this gave me the positive focus ahead of achieving something, and in turn inspiring others to follow my recipes and also enjoy eating a healthy diet. I am so grateful to everyone who kindly responded with positive feedback about my recipes, even recommending that I create my own cookbook.

I researched diets tirelessly, and I tried them all. I investigated the optimum blue zone healthy food diet choices, and from this, I learned to cook using raw and natural ingredients. I was inspired by Podcaster and Author Rich Roll, who had also collapsed age 39 years with ill health, and he had turned this life around by eating a vegan plant-based diet, and went on to become an Ultra Marathon Runner. He explained that "Plants are our healers".

I hadn't eaten meat or fish for the past seventeen years, since I became vegetarian aged twenty-four years, but I was unknowingly eating unhealthy processed 'candida (yeast) promoting' vegetarian food choices, or at times of very high stress 'no food choices'. Inspired by Rich Roll, I went from eating a highly processed, sugar fuelled western diet, to eating loads of plants, with no sugar, no gluten, no dairy, no processed foods, no alcohol... and initially what seemed like... no fun!

I learned that we are all individual when it comes to the subject of 'optimum' diet choices, but by eating a whole food plant-based diet, (and in my personal case; no meat), but adding wild caught fish and free-range eggs, is what worked, and continues to work for me.

I found giving up sugar extremely difficult, as I was very addicted to it. Now, I do not claim to be a saint with my diet transformation. There were times where my partner Mark and I went to the local superstore and emptied the shelves of chocolate easter eggs, and occasions where we fell into a cheesecake! The pleasure soon turning to pain and drowsiness, thereafter, further proving to us both, just how important our diet is to our health, but particularly with having ME and food sensitivities.

After eating, I often felt a sticky feeling inside my gut, and my partner Mark would routinely have to physically pull my arms and then my legs each day, to 'unstick' my insides and enable the drainage system in my stomach to work more efficiently. Mark said that he was "only pulling my leg!" So, I told him to "pull the other one!"

This gave me the idea to try removing all 'sticky food products', not just sugar, but also fruit and fructose and to replace them with healthy salts. I started including Dr Sarah Myhill's 'Sunshine salt' which contains the top 12 essential minerals. This change in my diet from sugar and yeast promoting foods to salt, helped to balance my gut microbiome, and change my internal environment from an acidic to an alkaline state. I found enormous improvements in my health, gut digestion, mobility and its efficiency from doing this.

Not everybody with ME has painful reactions to fruit, but I found that I had particularly bad reactions to citrus fruits (oranges and lemons), and so with continued healing ahead, I hope to be able to add fruits back into my diet in time.

Eating is a 'habitual routine' which can be changed, I discovered. Healthy Eating, is about creating new 'positive healthy eating daily routines' and feeling the rewards of our health, both physically and mentally. Most people have no idea how much better their day-to-day functionality could be, with positive and incremental healthy diet changes.

Our diet has a direct impact on all of of our daily functions, including one of the most important functions which is our ability to sleep deeply, which is absolutely 'essential' to ME patients, who cannot sleep properly, for we detoxify as we sleep.

Although some ME patients have found healing with 'The Perrin Technique' alone, I believe that for long term 'optimum health' and to reduce the chances of an ME relapse, or another health condition, our diet is absolutely quintessential in aiding recovery from any and all health conditions.

I found that a healthy whole food plant-based diet, with fish and eggs, provides the right nutrients and essential fats and vitamins which the body needs to function optimally. As Rich Roll says the plants (vegetables) are our healers, and I believe whatever our body is lacking in needs to be replenished. I completely changed my eating routine and diet choices. I swapped my traditional western breakfast choice of 'processed cereal with milk', to drinking an 'organic plant-based vegetable smoothie', packed with vitamins and minerals.

With a complete overhaul of my diet, I now genuinely crave vegetables instead of sugar, and the taste of eating 'real food' is exquisite and thoroughly satisfying, as it should be. My taste buds have come alive!

I now consistently listen to my gut in all things. I am grateful that I have what I call a 'superpower', where I have a severe allergic reaction to any food or drink products which are unhealthy. My body responds positively on both the 'inside and the outside', in eating this way. I have healthy skin, bright eyes and clearer vision, thicker sheen hair, strong nails, and best of all bright white teeth, without ever needing to see a dentist. My dentist did tell me years ago that if I don't eat any sugar, I most likely won't need to see him again, and he was right!

My nana once said "Eeh! Cathy, they didn't have 'organic' food in my day, they just called it food."

My nana was right, and she also said "Eeh! Cathy" a lot!

Even the natural plant-based food products that we eat today, are overloaded with pesticides and other toxic chemicals, which are now added to our soil and food produce, and are extremely harmful and toxic to our health, as well as to the soil and the worms needed to turn the soil within.

I now live 'The Good Life' and I grow my own food, and practise 'Organic Composting'. I have my own compost bin in the garden, and as I eat so many plants and vegetables, I fill up the compost bin daily, with peelings and leftovers. I also source local horse manure and rabbit droppings from friends who have animals, and add this to the compost bin, along with natural rainwater collected inside the garden water buts.

I do not drink any alcohol, and I dramatically increased my daily fluid intake of water to aid detoxification as I recovered, and water is now my main drink of choice. My kind-hearted friend Louisa Cornall recommended that I get a Berkey water filter with chlorine and fluoride filters, to help boost my health and my immune system.

As water is the most important and necessary fluid requirement for our survival, the Berkey water filter aids the removal of many toxic substances, chemicals and heavy metals, present within our drinking water. I personally believe that it is one of the best water filtration systems available. I explained to my dad "Did you know that our drinking water contains anti-depressants?

He replied "No wonder I'm so happy!".

We laughed.

I researched a wide range of healing food and drink products to help boost my immune system and detoxify my body.

One afternoon, I met two lovely ladies, Betty and Harriet, within the one-hundred-years-old Lancaster Atkinson's tea shop. We bonded instantly, and they kindly recommended a variety of Atkinson's tea choices that would help aid the detoxification of my system.

On hearing a little about my health condition and recovery journey, both ladies highlighted the incredible health benefits of drinking 'natural tea', over conventional tea bags, which can oftentimes be wrapped in plastic.

The ladies recommended that I try Ti Kwan Yin tea, for aiding detoxification of excess yeast in the gut, and also pointed out the benefits of the wide range of Atkinson's tea products they offered, including rosebud or camomile tea to aid sleep, peppermint or ginger and lemon tea for healing the gut, and mixed berries tea for mood enhancing benefits.

They also suggested how I could mix one or more teas together inside my Atkinson Tea Pot, indeed the combination of 'natural tea' benefits were endless.

Today, I drink Ti Kwan Yin and peppermint tea every morning, and my gut issues have healed dramatically thanks to a holistic approach to diet and fluid intake, in addition to 'The Perrin Technique' treatments.

From someone who 'didn't have time to eat' and did not enjoy cooking or eating food, I now truly love experimenting in the kitchen in creating, preparing, cooking and then eating 'real food'. Today I find that "Nothing tastes as good as wellness feels".

3. REST WITH ME

"When you feel bad… rest, when you feel good… rest" - Dr Raymond Perrin.

What I needed more than anything was 'rest'. I needed to completely rest both my mind and body.

In January 2014, I had jokingly begged for a year off work to sleep, and exactly one month later I learned to be careful what you wish for… As I was given ten years!

My ME symptoms were a combination of the seven dwarfs from the fairytale 'Sleeping beauty'. I was Sleepy, Sneezy, Dopey, Grumpy…and I had the stature to match!

I lived my life as a performer, a people pleaser, and a perfectionist, with not enough time in the day, and now I was suddenly forced to become a spectator, sedentary, and in solitude, with time appearing to last for an eternity. I now had all the time I had so desperately craved before, to focus on healing myself. For the first time in my life, I was advised to 'put myself first' and take care of myself the way I would take care of someone I loved.

In order to recover, I had to learn a brand-new way of living by activating the parasympathetic nervous system (the calm, rest and digest and healing mechanism) instead of the sympathetic nervous system (the excited, adrenalised, fight or flight mechanism).

For myself, and all who know me… this was going to be impossible. I got over excited at everything I did… including emptying a dishwasher! I lived out the proceeding years, in the main, either lying in bed or lying on the settee, and I found that this is a commonality with many severely affected ME patients.

Lying down with limited distractions to fill my days, I thankfully still managed to retain my 'laugh', and one of the funniest moments I watched play out on social media, was following an ME patient arguing with another ME patient. The first texting "Get back on the sofa!", with the retort "No! You get back on the sofa!" I cried laughing before falling asleep, and vowed that exchange was going into my 'stand-up comedy' show when I was better!

Every task, either mental or physical set me back. Each time I attempted to push through to do any task, my ME symptoms increased. I had to learn to say "No" to almost everything.

Saying "No" to well-meaning visitors was the hardest, because I wanted to see them, but every time they left, I crashed asleep in pain. I found that my healing was vastly improved and aided by being at rest in complete stillness and silence.

My rest included removing high stimuli devices such as mobile phone, TV and computers, anything that involved the use of the brain, which was of course everything!

If I had my recovery time again, I would stop and completely rest and not keep attempting any tasks, until I felt well enough to start gradually pacing activities, or when my healthcare provider agreed it, as the boom/bust cycle I was looped in, hugely compounded the longevity of my healing journey.

I was equipped with numerous support aids including a supportive mattress, shower stool, black out curtains, eye mask, and ear defenders.

I also found that, due to the shape of my flat upper spine, laying my head on two pillows, with a third pillow under the upper spine helped to support my back and neck during sleep, and this helped prevent my neck from subluxations, which had frequently occurred before.

I became aware that I was a 'mouth breather', because I couldn't breathe properly through my nose, likely after it was broken in childhood, and I had always taken 'sharp fast inhalations of breath' through my mouth.

I was recommended to try using Sterimar Baby Nasal Hygiene Salt Spray to aid decongestion. I emphasise here that the wording on the packet said for a 'baby'. The first time I used this baby spray up my nose, I passed out asleep from just one spray in each nostril, which highlights just how severely sick I was. However, I must add that this salt spray worked very successfully, and I continued to gradually use this, under medical guidance, over the proceeding months.

My partner Mark Singleton suggested that I start mouth taping, likely as a way to get me to stop talking!

He suggested that as I go to sleep, I tape a very small piece of micropore to the centre of the mouth, to help restore 'nasal breathing' and prevent 'mouth breathing'. Only applying enough micropore to the lips ensuring that I could still open and close my mouth, if I needed to during sleep.

I found that mouth taping was an excellent way to train my brain and body to breathe properly.

Nasal breathing enables a deeper inhalation of oxygen, and expands the lungs to a fuller capacity and consequently leads to deeper restorative sleep, with less sore and dry throats, from open mouth breathing on waking.

Now that the structural issues involving my jaw realignment were corrected through osteopathy with Dr Perrin, and my nasal passages were clear, I could actually breathe properly through my nose by day and by night, for the first time in my life. The rewards of being able to breathe properly are incredible, and essential to optimum health.

In the early stages of my recovery, I had no control whatsoever about when I slept, I would drift in and out of sleep by day and by night, and I found that forcing myself to try and stay awake made me even worse, so I decided to leave the healing process to nature. When I felt as though I needed a rest or I suddenly crashed asleep, I simply gave into it, and I took it. In the early to middle stages of recovery, I found that I could stay awake for slightly longer periods, but staying awake 'all day' simply wasn't possible for me, as I still crashed regularly, albeit for a lesser time period.

To aid the correction of the meridian cycle, I set myself a bedtime routine of 5pm to begin with, and whatever my crashes were by day, I stuck rigidly to this bedtime routine, like a small child in bedtime training. Having previously started my evening stage shows at 9pm, coupled with a six-hour round trip, my meridian cycle was completely off.

Throughout my life, I had always found a lot of difficulty in getting to sleep at night, and then struggled sleeping through the nights, often enduring terrifying nightmares, irritable bladder, and anaphylactic choking episodes in my sleep, where at times I was very worried I may not rouse.

As such, it took me quite long while of this new 'sleep training' routine, before I could fall asleep and stay asleep long enough to feel refreshed the following day. Over the years, as I continued to detoxify, I found that I could gradually stay awake longer and longer throughout the day, and the very first time I stayed awake with ease until 9pm was a huge milestone!

As I gradually recovered, my awake and sleep cycle corrected itself, and I slept deeply undisturbed throughout the night, a brand-new experience for me, and this aided the restoration of my health enormously.

I can now sleep deeply, and my mind and my emotional state are calm and balanced.

4. PACING WITH ME:

"Only do half of what you feel capable of doing. Stick to the fifty percent rule." Dr Raymond Perrin.

As a high achiever, I failed miserably in the early stages of my recovery journey, in following Dr Perrin's 'fifty percent rule', because I had previously been so highly physically active, my version of 50 percent was actually another person's 100 percent!

I found that once I started any physical or mental task, 'I couldn't stop, not wouldn't stop'. My brain was so high wired, and full of toxins, that I genuinely couldn't stop...until I dropped. There were numerous occasions where I excitedly professed to Dr Perrin that I was "suddenly cured!" Only to find that an hour later, I had crashed again.

One afternoon, I was trying to push myself to carry a light shopping basket into Asda, when my legs suddenly collapsed and I couldn't walk. I asked a young member of staff could he please assist me, and he refused. I looked up at him and I said, "But your badge says 'Happy to help!'"

I hadn't realised how taxing that mental exertion is on our recovery, and not just physical exertion. Although I believed I was resting, in lying on the settee, I was still using my brain, and I had to learn to stop reading for example, and come off social media, as this required a very high level of mental energy in constantly thinking and using high stimuli electronic devices.

Dr Perrin knew **my personality very well, having treated so many Type 'A' personality patients, all stuck in the boom or bust cycle,** so in the end, he instructed me to do "Absolutely nothing". My homework was to "Stop thinking."

I am grateful to have had care support provided by wonderful professional carers over the years, including Penny and Gemma in the early stages of my ill health, and later my full-time carer was Lisa Kirkby. The care support I received was absolutely essential to my recovery, because I had previously always done everything myself, and I learned that with ME "It's not what you do, it's what happens after you've done it."

This rest and pacing balance was something that I had been fighting against, and thanks to the care support in place, I was able to give in to the pacing ritual, and the boom-bust cycle, and stop absolutely everything, and completely rest both mind and body. In the end my body thanked me for it.

Over time, through detoxification, I gradually learned to tune in and listen to my body, and I was better able to control my ability to start Pacing and only do half any physical or mental activity. This was one of the most difficult adjustments for me. Learning to 'give in' without 'giving up'.

My carer, Lisa, helped me with so much over many years, and her level of compassion and care as well as her sense of humour, positively encouraged me throughout. My carer, Penny, was also incredibly compassionate and supportive to my needs, and she bought me a keyring which read 'Never give up'. This is a gift I treasure with words that I will stand by forever...now that I can stand!

5. TALK TO ME:
"Issues are like tissues. You pull one out and another appears!" - Gary Goldstein.

Talking therapy with the right therapist for you can be extremely valuable to 'everyone'. However, talking therapy is not a cure for a physical condition such as ME, and I campaigned through Parliament to have CBT and GET removed from the NHS NICE guidelines as recommended treatments for ME.

In the early stages of my condition, I was so sick that I couldn't physically talk, so my entire focus was on my physical recovery.

However, over time, I found that being able to talk to someone, was particularly helpful in coping with this sudden onset of a physically overwhelming, and debilitatingly painful health condition. At this time, I found person centred counselling most supportive, as I was given the space to talk freely.

I also tried a number of holistic therapies which I found particularly supportive, all of which engaged the parasympathetic nervous system needed to rest and heal.

These included hypnotherapy, meditation, and emotional-somatic release the latter being administered by my partner Mark Singleton and Ana Paula Bianchi who are both qualified 'Perrin Technique Practitioners'.

Mark and Ana, who met at The Upledger Institute whilst training in advanced craniosacral therapy, performed a dual healing treatment therapy called 'Somato Emotional Release'. This combined craniosacral therapy, massage therapy, and talking therapy.

Lying down, in therapy with one practitioner holding my head, and feeling for the cranio sacral rhythm, the second practitioner listened into the body and gently moved my arms and legs releasing any tightness or constriction inside. The second practitioner then talked to me and asked questions about any potential traumas I may wish to release into the sacred space.

I found the emotional somatic release treatment extremely beneficial to my health, as it freed up any tightness in my body, aided the function of the drainage of the lymphatic system, whilst also releasing any blocked traumas from my mind.

At one point, Ana and Mark were both holding my outstretched arms and gently pulling and unblocking any constrictions I felt inside. This was the benefit of the dual therapy treatment. I asked if this position was called the 'Jesus release' which brought much resounding laughter, to end the session.

I was blessed to have had therapeutic support from various professionals and friends, and I shall continue to use these therapies in future.

I personally found complete healing from my 'emotional traumas' came from contacting the Ministry of Justice in 2016, and reporting all the criminal offences against me.

DI David Groombridge from the Lancashire Constabulary came to my home, as I was housebound. Here, DI Groombridge gave me the time and space I needed to report all of my assaults, which included two drugging assaults against me. This took many months due to the severity of my health condition. DI

Groombridge handled my situation with the utmost professionalism, care and support throughout, and over time justice was done. Three arrests were made, with criminal charges brought against them. One offender was imprisoned. DI Groombridge encouraged me to write this book. He said that if my story helps to save just one life, then it will be worth it. I was saddened to hear that he had passed away in 2020, and I thank him for his invaluable support.

After I had successfully reported all of my traumas, my mind felt freed, but my physical health didn't improve, confirming that ME is not psychological.

I needed a manual 'treatment' for the severity level of my physical health condition ME, especially with having chemical overload from multiple highly toxic chemicals, and for this I used 'The Perrin Technique'.

6. DETOX WITH ME:
"If a fish is sick, what do you do, inject the fish, or change its environment?" - Dr Robert Young.

In 2016, as I began to detoxify myself with 'The Perrin Technique' treatments, my diet, and other healing modalities, I began to 'detoxify my world'. Due to having had carbon monoxide poisoning, and high paint fumes exposure inside my home, I desperately needed oxygen.

After the plumber found a broken flue pipe emitting carbon monoxide in my kitchen, I had further health and safety checks done within my home, including a visit from the local 'Preston Fire Service' who installed carbon monoxide detectors throughout.

I also had an EnviroVent ventilation unit installed, and this pumped air 24/7 throughout the house. I was advised by the technician to open both the front and back windows of my property daily to circulate fresh air at all times, when possible. Further environmental checks found lead pipes directly feeding my water supply, and damp on certain internal walls. Gas checks were safely passed, and I now have regular health and safety checks and services of household appliances.

One afternoon, I got a large bin liner, and I filled it with everything highly toxic from both the inside and the outside of my home. With a co-morbidity of 'Mast Cell Activation Syndrome', where my face and body flared up when using any toxic products, I replaced all the highly chemical laden products, with as natural as possible alternatives. Indeed, removing all of these highly toxic chemicals from my world, has massively reduced my overall symptoms.

I found my dream all-purpose medicinal product to be coconut oil. This is now my daily multi-use product of choice. I eat it, use it for cooking, cleaning my teeth, as a daily face and body cream, a hair treatment, as my Perrin massage treatment oil, as a wound healing ointment, and I even feed it my little dog Tinker for health benefits for us both.

I wanted to purify the air within my home, so I filled my home with indoor plants including The Peace Lily, Spider plants, the Snake plant:

(Sansevieria Trifasciata), Aloe Vera, and Bromeliad. I also got an Air Conditioning Unit as I was struggling to breathe, and this became hugely supportive during my recovery.

As I detoxified my home, I used this opportunity of having infinite time in the days, to clear out lots of things within my home which I had accumulated over the years from working non-stop. Although I was obsessively neat and tidy, there was a lot!

I had carer support with this, as this was a particularly difficult task with having limited cognitive and physical function, but I found that the rewards were great and incredibly cathartic. Like clearing out the nest and making a fresh start, it was 'out with the old life' and 'in with the new'.

I had accumulated a garage full of drama props, costumes and homemade set pieces and sat at the very top of all this was a huge blow-up whale! Over many months we sent many boxes to charity, local schools and theatre schools who were excited to include these in their classes. My favourite moment was waving off my friend Roz Dunning, as she had kindly collected some props to give to a local theatre school, and she held on tight to the huge whale head sticking out of the car window. I had become quite attached to that whale, and I likened this moment to waving goodbye to your child going off to university!

One day, I decided that I was going to get to the bottom of my ME, and as such, I was recommended to have colonic treatment with Lynne McDougall. Lynne is so genuine and kind-hearted, and she made me feel completely at ease in her care.

After a number of standard colonics, Lynne asked "Cathy, would you like a coffee enema?"

"No thank you" I quipped "I don't drink coffee!"

"It's not to drink." Lynne laughingly replied, by now knowing my sense of humour.

"At what point do I ask for milk and two sugars?" I continued.

Laughter.

I found overall health and gut improvements from Lynne's colonic treatments, and I would certainly go again in the future.

As well as removing chemical stressors on my system, I also found that I needed to remove emotional stressors too.

With having ME, I couldn't physically cope with any additional stressors. When I was in highly emotionally stressful situations, both positive or negative, my physical symptoms increased. My nervous system jacked, my legs would collapse, and I would experience right arm tremors.

I found that any toxic and negative energy was so overwhelming to my system, that I had to remove myself physically and mentally from certain people and certain situations, in order to have the very best chance to recover.

Whereas healthy people can get emotional, and then carry on with their lives as normal, I found that I would be physically wiped out for days, or indeed months, following a negative interaction.

Dr Perrin explained to me that stress of any kind in ME patients is harmful for it over-stimulates the sympathetic nervous system. During recovery from ME emotional stress needs to be avoided as much as possible, whilst the system heals.

Every time I went against a gut feeling from within and I didn't listen to my gut, I suffered overwhelming physical symptoms. This became a warning sign for me in all aspects of my life, to tune into myself, and know that "If something doesn't feel right, then it isn't right for ME."

I found stepping away from stressors in order to take the necessary time to heal was very rewarding, and once my system was operating in the parasympathetic instead of the sympathetic, I could more easily cope with both good and bad stress, without any increase in my symptoms. I regularly remind myself that everyone is on their own life journey, and oftentimes our behaviour is unconscious. I set up healthy boundaries with people, and invited more people who aligned with me into my life, for a peaceful life journey.

Here in a place of inner peace, I can better understand that nothing is ever personal, 'Hurt people hurt people'. I now practice removing myself from negative situations, and I think to myself "Thank you for showing me who you are."

As we detox our world, we open up a brand-new chapter in our life, and we start to attract other 'like-minded souls' with the same core values, and we realise that we can choose precisely who we want in our lives.

I am not perfect, but the best thing is, I no longer try to be. I accept myself exactly as I am today, and I try to do the best with the tools that I have been given.

I found extremely positive rewards from this complete detoxification of the world around me, it gave a time for self-reflection, promoted positive self-worth, and it aided my healing from within.

7. MEDITATE WITH ME:
"Your life will not be measured by what you took out but by what you had to give." - Guy Burgs 'The Art of Meditation'.

I found an incredible way to aid my recovery was in practising the daily art of meditation. Living with ME, particularly in the bed bound and housebound stages, brought feelings of loneliness and isolation, being stuck inside a body which is unable to physically do things it once could. The resting and healing process, presented me with an enormous amount of time inside my mind.

I found meditation helped to strengthen and empower my mindset. I used it for pain management, and it also gave me a manageable task to do each day. I learned that we cannot escape negative energy, but we can train our minds and bodies not to react to it through practicing meditation. I lived my life surrounded by noise. Nonstop music, singing, dancing and entertaining. I would never walk anywhere without having music playing inside my headphones. I chose holiday destinations with upbeat music playing, and activities constantly surrounding me to participate in. Where I was once afraid of the sound of silence, the silence now became my best friend and my ultimate healer.

My head was so busy and noisy that I initially struggled to 'meditate' for even a few minutes, I couldn't find the stillness within, as my rest time had previously been a Zumba dance class! Like changing my diet, learning to meditate was about removing old unhelpful patterns and lifestyle choices and introducing new positive ones.

I first started mediation using an app called 'Headspace' which is a guided spoken meditation that teaches you how to meditate, and I used this regularly in the early stages, and I found this very helpful. Over time, I could meditate for 30 minutes which had at first seemed like a lifetime!

As I progressed in my own ability to meditate, I soon realised this practice needed to be done in complete silence. I started learning meditation with the incredible Guy Burgs, the founder and chief tutor of the 'Art of Meditation'. Guy's meditations are a mixture of guided and self-reflective meditations, as well as incorporating integral moments of silence and stillness. Guy's meditations encourage us to let go and do absolutely nothing, and allow the process to happen, rather than push through to find the answers.

Today, I always feel a sense of complete inner peace and calm after practising with Guy, and I hope to attend a meditation workshop with him in person in the future, as my partner Mark Singleton has had the pleasure of doing.

Over time, I trained myself to meditate for hours, in complete silence. Meditation is a tool which I practise daily, every morning on waking, and every evening to aid a deeper sleep. I have a meditation 'present mind' cushion, to sit on in front of a meditation statue, acting as a symbolic prayer temple on my dresser. I find having a physical mediation focus ahead can also be very cathartic and healing.

It is also very healing with having ME, to reduce visual stimuli and either meditate looking out into space, or with eyes closed to focus more deeply on the breath. Lying down, or seated, I focus on the breath, and with my hands gently rested on my stomach, I inhale deeply into the lower abdomen, bringing 'positive energy' and I then exhale longer lengths of breath to detox 'negative energy'.

I find outdoor meditation amongst the trees and nature exceptionally rewarding and healing on multiple levels; including increasing oxygen, peace, quiet and stillness, and in being away from electricity. I now sit down with my back against a tree, or on a tree stump looking out into the abyss for at least 10-30 minutes whilst focusing on the breath. Meditation is so healing for us as well as for our pets. I would sit my little dog Tinker on my knee, and he would become very still and peaceful, as all animals are acutely sensitive to peaceful surrounds and nature.

However, I do wish to recommend choosing the right places for this, as I was once stood by a tree mediating, when I overheard a lady behind me say to her daughter in a very strong northern accent; "Ooh! we are not going down there, there's a lady stood by a tree waiting for sex!" This interrupted my mediation, and

I couldn't stop laughing. After this incident I vowed only to choose private wood land areas to mediate, instead of public parks!

8. GROUND AND PROTECT ME:
"The greatest oak was once a little nut who held its ground." - Author Unknown.

I was additionally suffering from severe 'Electro Magnetic Sensitivity' (EMS). Whenever I used any electronic technology, it caused severe reactions, including a headache, a metallic taste in my mouth, burning pain in both my fingers and inside my eyes, tinnitus, and breathing issues. I would frequently drop my burning hot mobile phone, as though it was a hot potato. I would also feel dizzy and collapse in places with high levels of electricity, wifi, ultraviolet lights, or loud music.

At times, when I hugged someone, including my little dog Tinker, I would see a spark of bright electricity light, and literally electrocute us both! That travelling circus was beaconing! The EMS was particularly apparent during storms. I was so sensitive, that I could feel a pressure inside my head before the storm was actually present. Then as the storm began, I felt like I was 'electrocuting', as Danny describes in the musical 'Grease'... it was "Electrifying!".

In 2015, I purchased a grounding sheet for my bed. This was a Groundology bed sheet which plugs into the wall socket and purportedly helps de-charge the nervous system during sleep. The bed sheets are 100% organic cotton, with conductive silver fibres woven through the material which connect to the Earth's natural energy in order to improve sleep quality, reduce inflammation and provide an overall enhancement of wellbeing.

I found that my initial detox was so severe, that my bedsheet turned black and it had to be thrown away, and as such I would recommend laying on an old sheet in the initial stages, so as not to damage the Groundology bed sheet.

Dr Perrin advised that during storms I should 'ground myself' on a non-carpeted floor, and wear EMS protective headwear. I was visited by a kind-hearted community safety advisor Keith Bridge, from 'Preston Fire Station'. He believed that my EMS symptoms were genuine, and he was very empathetic to my health situation.

Keith suggested that I try using an aluminium foil blanket, which would normally be used for keeping people warm after running a marathon, or after being pulled out of a river, but in my case, it might give 'radio magnetic protection'. I followed both Dr Perrin and Keith's advice, and these were an enormous support to me. They acted as a barrier to the electricity charge. My symptoms reduced, and I could finally go to sleep at night.

My little dog Tinker would also benefit from the aluminium foil blanket. During storms he would squeak in distress and spin in circles on the bed next to me, sometimes falling off the bed. When I covered us both in the blanket, he calmed down and fell straight asleep. I knew then, that my EMS was a physical symptom, as it was happening to us both. An electrician also visited my home and he grounded all my electrics, switched off my Wi-Fi and hard wired the house, and my EMS symptoms reduced significantly.

As I was practising Meditation within nature, I also began practising Tree hugging and sitting in nature amongst the trees to ground myself from the electrical frequencies I was experiencing, and this was an enormous health support, as the trees were helping to 'ground me'.

I was recommended to try having Himalayan salt lamps throughout my home, and particularly by my bed, as they are claimed to be 'natural ionisers' and change the electrical charge of the circulating air, as well as improving the air quality. Himalayan salt lamps also have mood and sleep enhancing beneficial claims, and these claims are based on the ancient practise of 'halotherapy'.

Every night I now practise turning the Himalayan salt lamp on, whilst placing Himalayan salt pieces in a line from the top of my chest down to my stomach as I meditate, and these all-aid relaxation and help support a deeper sleep.

9. WALK WITH ME:
"It does not matter how slow you go, so long as you do not stop!" Confucious.

Remembering the story of 'The tortoise and the hare', I reminded myself throughout my healing journey that the tortoise won the race. I was healing from a disease that didn't exist, and that also had no cure. I knew that if I stayed sick, I would be believed by the ME community, but not all of the medical community, but I also knew that if one day I recovered, that some of the ME community may never believe that I was ever that sick to begin with.

I detoxed and I rested, and I paced, and in time I could walk a short distance without experiencing Post Exertion Malaise (PEM).

I remembered that "ME is not what we do today, it's what happens to us tomorrow."

Over time, tomorrow's post exercise pain never came, which was both incredible and unbelievable. I began to walk a very short distance every day around the garden, and I gradually built up over the years to travel further distances, constantly working within my pacing routine parameters following Dr Perrin's 'fifty per cent rule'.

I also tried Tai Chi as my partner was an instructor. I learned how to stand, arms by my side with centralised posture looking ahead into the distance. At first this was looking outside of my bedroom window, and over time this was looking out into the woods. Tai chi was excellent for aiding my balance issues from vestibular inner ear damage, as well as complimenting the breath work I was doing, and I combined this with meditation.

I also began very basic gentle Yoga stretches on a yoga mat in the home. Gently rolling side to side across the mat to massage the kidneys and lower back, and gentle yoga stretches and positions which didn't hyper extend my body and joints.

217

I now 'play the xylophone' on my spine each day by gently releasing it vertebrae by vertebrae, something that was impossible before, as it was previously very tight and constricted.

Tia Chi, Yoga and gentle walking all activate the 'parasympathetic nervous system', whilst jogging, weightlifting, dancing and other strenuous exercise activities, activate the 'sympathetics' which we now understand are an issue in ME. The rewards of engaging the parasympathetic nervous system through gentle exercise, after a lifetime of 'sympathetic overload' through vigorous exercise is so healing.

I used to be the 'hare' running everywhere, around the block, in the gym, up the stairs, and never ever having enough time in the day, 'always racing through life and missing the view'. Now as the 'tortoise', I can walk alone in silence and feel completely at peace, enjoying the view and taking in the surrounds, the shapes, the colours and textures and the beauty of this world of which I had been missing.

By slowing down everything, this helps to heal the overstimulated nervous system and the busy mind, allowing inner peace and healing within, which can ensue for a lifetime.

10. CREATE WITH ME:
"Same world different view." - Catherine Vandome.

In order to heal from anything, we first need to find a 'purpose'. Lying in bed unable to turn my head on the pillow, I closed my eyes and prayed that if someone could please come and save me, I would spend the rest of my life thanking them… and that someone was Dr Perrin. I knew from very early on in my own recovery journey, that I wanted to try to help save other peoples' lives from living with ME, and that became my purpose and my mission.

As I began to recover, I was inspired by a book called 'The Artists Way' by Julia Cameron, and this book was an invaluable recovery tool within my healing process. I took from the book a most valuable healing modality of 'Journaling' in writing 3 pages of A4 every morning, called 'Morning pages'.

Every day I would write a 'stream of consciousness' journal no more or less than 3 pages of A4, and I wrote down absolutely everything that I felt, or wanted, or hoped for, onto the page as per Julia Cameron's creative instructions.

The idea behind the journaling being that if we write down and express everything, including our thoughts and anxieties onto the page daily, that this would reduce the level of anxiety or stress or worries we hold within our nervous system.

In the same way that Antonin Artaud's 'Theatre of Cruelty' is a therapeutic way of bearing one's soul and releasing desires and emotions into the theatre space, as a form of cathartic release. In journaling our innermost emotions are released onto the page, and we have the freedom of expression and complete privacy needed to write anything we wish to, without judgement. This process was life changing for me, and is one of the best healing modalities I have adapted and one which I still use today.

When we use a pen and paper to write, we are forced to slow down, and we can then engage our logical, questioning and creative thinking brain and we can more easily think and solve problems for ourselves. Whereas when we type, in using our phones and computers, we tend to become more formal and structured in our pattern of thinking, in staring at the screen, without having the time and space for an inner dialogue and using our own 'independent thinking'.

Handwriting through journaling also provides complete privacy, and an enhanced state of peace away from EMF's, as well as developing a uniqueness and individuality in our own style of handwriting and creative ways of expression.

In doing so, we get the necessary time alone in the peace and quiet to contemplate and reflect, which we rarely get the opportunity to do with the business mode and speed of typing words into a computer. I started writing (mostly backwards and inaudibly at first), and I continued to keep daily journals every day over the years, until I was feeling well enough to read them back, without becoming too distressed by them.

I highly recommend journaling, firstly for a cathartic release, where I found that I could take control of my own life, and become my own therapist at home, for nobody truly understands you better than you do. I found that journaling works in tandem with talking therapy, where I could release private thoughts and emotions onto the page post therapy, or after being in a stressful situation, as well as within my daily morning (or evening) pages routine. These two modalities work hand in glove.

Journaling also helps with the ME healing process, by aiding my brain to repair in using thinking and writing skills, which over time helped to restore my brains overall cognitive function. After a lifetime of high energy activities, I started to develop peaceful, creative and artistic passions once lost in childhood, which is indeed the purpose of *The Artist Way* book.

I could no longer do my old creative activities in dancing, singing, acting or playing the drums, so *The Artists Way* book encouraged me to find my new purpose in expressing myself through other creative and artistic forms.

These new creative activities included writing, drawing, painting, therapy, meditation and blogging. All my old creative activities engaged the sympathetic nervous system, whilst these new creative activities stimulated the 'parasympathetic nervous system'. In the early stages of my recovery, even doing peaceful creative activities utilised so much energy, with having ME. That was where the Pacing came in useful, which was set by myself, and ensured that I had small set times to do particular tasks, without pushing through and crashing afterwards.

Alongside campaigning, I also set up a support group and a website for ME patients globally, and on good days I shared all the healing modalities which were helping me. By connecting with the outside world, I no longer felt alone with ME, and each day had a purpose. Most importantly, the process of journaling for myself, turned into a book. This book. I even thought of the title of this book back in 2016, where I found that I had written inside my journal "I am going to write a book and help save lives and it's going to be called 'The truth about ME." This became my life's blueprint.

In 2024, I started reading through all the years of my journals, which was a particularly difficult part of the healing journey for me, as I had lost a great deal of memory over the years, and I was now reading things that I had absolutely no recollection of writing. However, it was a very emotional and cathartic healing experience, as I wanted to get rid of anything negative which I had endured, as a form of letting go of the past and entering a new world.

I got a huge bin liner and shredded the private diaries page by page, whilst retaining a new journal of inspiring quotes and thoughts from the past ten years, which were of particular significance to me. I then collected the large bags of hand shredded journals, and with support from my partner Mark Singleton, I put them into a large paper burner and ceremoniously burned them, letting go of the past ten years of sickness and trauma.

A week later I found my book publisher. It happened at the right time in my healing journey. I truly believe that everything happens for a reason, although we often cannot see it at the time. One of the most rewarding things I did, was to free flow and write out my entire life story filled with the good, the bad and the ugly, all of it out in full. I started at the beginning of my life, and I flooded the page with all the memories of everything that I had gone through, and I found this extremely cathartic.

Over time, as I healed, I was able to return to the beginning of my life again, and rewrite my whole story, no longer traumatised by particular events, and as such, I no longer felt the need to include them.

This time in writing, I saw the comedy in the tragedy, and I could now remember with increased clarity the finite detail within all the positive life experiences which I have had. Now in rewriting everything out again in a different format, I was inspired to turn my life story into this book.

I want to encourage everybody thinking of doing so, to write a book. To help you to start writing a book remember that all you need to do is to 'write your first line', and to help anyone who has started a book and cannot finish it, then all you need to do is remember your books 'purpose' and 'blueprint' (your life's plan). The past ten years has been both the worst, and yet the best thing to have ever happened to me. I have seen the truth in myself and those around me, and I am so blessed to have had the support I have been given in order to heal.

I am so grateful for all the little things in life, things I once took for granted. Everyday matters. Every minute counts. Every moment is precious, and 'Life Is Beautiful'…which also happens to be my favourite film.

I have many creative ideas and projects I hope to realise ahead, and I am so excited about my future. I am now functioning each day from a place of peace and healing in listening to my gut, and that will ensure I maintain the balance in all things needed for optimum functioning.

My advice to all ME patients who are bed bound or housebound is to never give up hope, use this precious gift of time to reignite an old passion, or find a brand-new purpose, and the rewards will be bountiful. Though we may be bed or housebound, we are bound only by the limitations with which we set ourselves. I share my journey and healing modalities so that you too may have the very best chance to recover. Some patients may need one or two of the healing modalities, I needed all the above.

For the first time in my life, I learned that my life matters too. Life is about helping each other, and as Dr Perrin and others have helped me, so I hope to pay it forwards and help you. Above all always remember that laughter is the best medicine. Try to find the comedy in the tragedy, and keep following the bright light ahead as you navigate your way through the heavily wooded area and into the light. After ten years by my side, my little companion dog, Tinker has taught me very simple core life values; 'love deeply, rest frequently, trump freely, be there for each other always, and above all find the joy in everything, by getting very, very excited and spinning in a circle at the simplest of life's activities, such as eating your breakfast!'

My recovery strategy is simple "Trust in the healing process. Believe in yourself. Forgive everybody everything. Be free and happy and do good always. Speak only your truth. Stand up for yourself. Make positive changes to your life and the lives of others in all you do. Help others always, as this brings the greatest rewards in life. Above all be the example you wish others to be."

When we are no longer here, people will only recall whether we were a good person, they will not remember what job we had, or how big our house was, they will only remember the size of our heart, and that love starts with ourselves as we heal from within. It is time to live your best life, filled with self-love, self-care, and inner peace. You are a truly 'Magnanimous Empath'.

"Speak your truth and only your truth. Don't get distracted by those who are committing wrong doings, people will see this in time. Instead focus all your positive energy on promoting the good of your own mission, which is to help save lives and help others to gain access to 'The Perrin Technique' by Dr Raymond Perrin."
Buddhist Monk Friend

CHAPTER TWENTY-FOUR: YOU Inspire ME
Holding out for a Hero. Never give up on ME!

"We cannot change the cards we are dealt, just how we play the hand." - Randy Pausch.

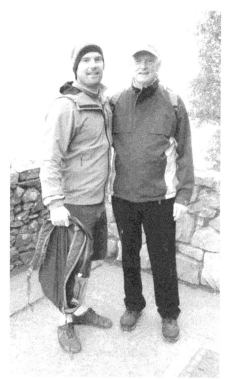

Catherine Vandome's partner Mark Singleton - 'The Perrin Technique' Practitioner at The Fulwood Therapy Centre, with his father James Singleton - Head of Clinical Psychology and Consultant Clinical Psychologist at Royal Preston Hospital (retd and recently deceased), in 2019.

The final chapter of my book is dedicated to my kind-hearted, loving and caring partner Mark Singleton, and in loving memory of his patient, loyal and wise father James Singleton.

> *My son Mark (The Author's partner) returned suddenly from Australia. After taking his degree he arranged a tour around the Far East, with two of his university friends. He was very down and had no energy. This was not the son whom I had seen over the years.*
> *As a child, Mark has always been lively, assertive and outgoing. He was also strong minded and quick to make friends. From this lively adventurous young man, he was now down, depressed and completely lacking in energy.*

After talking things over with him, and knowing his background, I realised that although he was presenting as depressed, the depression appeared to be a product of his severe lack of energy.

As a clinical psychologist who had worked for decades in adult mental health, I was very saddened to find that I could not help my son. I realised that what he was suffering from was physiological and not psychological.

This realisation was confirmed in 1999 when Mark was diagnosed with ME/Chronic Fatigue Syndrome by Dr Wendy Denning at 'The Integrated Medical Centre' in London. Dr Denning is a General Practitioner specialising in ME/Chronic Fatigue Syndrome.

Over the decades of having this chronic illness, my son Mark has tried many different approaches to aid his recovery, without success.

In 2016, Mark started treatment with Dr Raymond Perrin at the Perrin Clinic in Prestwich, near Manchester. Fortunately, as a result of this treatment, Mark is slowly but surely improving. I believe that 'The Perrin Technique' is the way forward.

James Singleton - BSc, Dip Psych, C Psychol, AFBPs) - Head of Clinical Psychology and Consultant Clinical Psychologist at Royal Preston Hospital (retd and recently deceased)

It was love at first sight…so he tells me! My memory is severely impaired. Mark Singleton picked me up at a funeral, literally, and carried me on his back thereafter, until Dr Perrin explained why he shouldn't do this with ME, as patients need to protect the spine.

"Don't lift anything heavy." Dr Perrin instructed

'Well Cathy's only seven stone!" Mark replied.

Our first date at Lytham Prom was like a 'Little Britain' sketch, with me flopped over the side of a wheelchair professing "I'm Jessie J!" Mark not knowing anything about my career history, accepting that I might well be delusional. There were moments I'm sure that Mark pushed me in a wheelchair at Lytham prom by the sea, and had to resist the urge to keep pushing!

I was so poorly, that Mark didn't tell me that he also had ME, as he didn't want to worry me. He waited until I was in better health before he shared his own story with me. I can honestly say that without the love and support from my partner Mark, I may not have made it this far. Mark believed me, and he supported me physically and emotionally throughout, and he literally carried me back to full health. We laughed through the darkest moments in both of our recovery journeys under Dr Perrin.

I am honoured to have met and fallen in love with such a kind-hearted, genuine, and caring man as Mark, with all of his fathers' qualities, both of whom devoted their entire life to helping others, and Mark was doing so at the same time as being in pursuit of healing himself. Here is Marks story, he is now a qualified 'Perrin Technique Practitioner', and helping others to heal from ME.

Mark Singleton's Story: (Author's partner)

I first started with the symptoms of ME/CFS in my late teens. On reflection these symptoms crept up on me, with good days and bad days.

After a holiday in Greece, at the age of twenty, I was so ill and dehydrated that I couldn't keep up with the pace of my friends.

On returning to the UK my symptoms persisted. After several weeks I went to see my GP and complained of feeling constantly tired. My doctor told me that it was probably a virus. At the time I did not know that this was 'doctor's code' for "I don't know what's wrong with you."

The symptoms continued and I was feeling tired all the time, despite having a large amount of rest. It felt as though I was constantly hung over without actually having had a drink.

Throughout my final year at Manchester University, my ill health continued. I mentioned to my friends how tired I was, but after the fatigue continued for several months, I didn't want to complain anymore, because who wants to hear that?

I assumed and hoped that this exhaustion was related to a student lifestyle and that a healthier lifestyle would bring my energy levels back.

After graduating, I planned to travel around the world, and so I got a job in a bar working over fifty hours per week. I was also exercising and eating healthily. Some days I was up at 7am. I would cycle to work in a restaurant bar in the morning, at 3pm I would run three miles to the gym and weight train, then get a lift back to work, complete a late bar work shift, and then cycle home afterwards at approximately 11.30pm.

I believed that I could push through to health by sheer force of will, but I was wrong. To my utter dismay, my ME/CFS symptoms worsened with neck tension and pain, and a huge degree of brain fog.

Being in what other people would describe as 'good shape' with my symptoms still worsening, I concluded that this must be 'all in the mind'. A common misconception about ME/CFS in the 1990's, and unfortunately still to this day. I saw the tiredness as a sign of weakness and became depressed, as I began to believe that I would never recover.

I was prescribed a number of different anti-depressants and reluctantly took them for several weeks, although none of the medication had a positive impact on my ME/CFS symptoms or my depression. I told my parents how I was feeling and they supported me in looking for 'alternative' treatments.

By the age of twenty-four, I was looking and feeling more and more run down. I was only well enough to pursue part time work as a waiter in a restaurant, which didn't relate at all to my Economics degree.

I researched my health and found out about a clinic in London that combined conventional medicine with complimentary practices. I arranged an appointment at the clinic with a doctor who diagnosed me with Chronic Fatigue Syndrome (CFS).

This doctor also arranged a hair mineral analysis and the results came back saying that my mineral balance was very out of kilter. I had an excess of particular heavy metals and a lack of certain essential minerals.

This gave me some evidence that my state of ill health was not 'all in my mind' and gave the doctor a plan of action for me. I was prescribed melatonin for sleep, plus a liquid mineral supplement and a sugar and dairy free diet to follow.

I returned home and followed the doctor's advice. Over the next few months my symptoms decreased a little, but the tiredness continued.

Over the next few years, I tried various other alternative/complimentary treatments in the hope of recovery, but to little effect. I tried conventional massage, reflexology, homeopathy, acupuncture and various other diet and supplement protocols.

I also tried person centred counselling, which did help the level of depression I was experiencing, but did nothing for my ME/CFS symptoms. I also read numerous health books trying to find some relief from my symptoms.

At age twenty-five, I stumbled upon a book called 'Chi Gung'' by Daniel Reid, and browsing through the book in store, I realised that it was about gaining energy, and I thought "Well I need energy, perhaps this can help?". I started practising the exercises in the book, and after further research I found a good Chi Gung and Tai Chi Instructor.

This practise had positive effects in improving my circulation, and took the aches and pains away, which I was feeling on waking every morning. The benefits of this practise have been so useful that I have practised this every day from that day.

This practise has cured the Raynaud's on my toes which used to be blue/white even in a warm bath. However, I still had problems with my energy levels, such that I wasn't capable of working a full-time job.

In my late 20's, I resigned myself to my illness, believing that I may find things that help, but that I would never truly get better.

I remained in this situation for over a decade, monitoring my energy expenditure. I did not explain to people that I had ME/CFS, as frankly I was ashamed to be lacking in energy, and I believed that they would think that it was 'all in my head'.

I was always pushing to do as much as my body would allow, sometimes overdoing it and needing even more rest.

At times my diet was very healthy for months on end, with natural foods and no processed foods or sugar, and I definitely noticed the benefits when this was the case, but I was still not recovering from my condition.

At times, in frustration, I would say "To hell with it! I am never going to get better so what's the point?" I would then eat sugary processed foods that left me feeling considerably worse.

I lived a life waking up feeling battered, like being hung over and having the flu, struggling to think and find words, and unable to trust that I can get through a regular day with the lack of energy I had. I was at night going to sleep with the nerves in my neck and back burning and tense.

In medical terms I endured; chronic fatigue, brain fog, memory difficulties, disrupted sleep, night sweats, neck stomach and joint pain, and the need to sleep intermittently throughout the day for two decades.

Finally, at the age of forty, my supportive girlfriend Cathy, (The Author of this book), persuaded me to go and see Neuroscientist and Osteopath Dr Raymond Perrin.

At this point in my life, I had done a great deal of research around my health, and I had become somewhat jaded towards anybody offering a treatment for ME/CFS.

In fact, I had previously read Dr Perrin's book 'The Perrin Technique' many years before, but had dismissed it, along with other books claiming to treat 'or cure' CFS/ME.

In 2016, it was with much scepticism that I stepped into Dr Raymond Perrin's office, inside 'The Perrin Clinic' in Prestwich.

In a short space of time, I realised that this was a kind, intelligent and decent man, who genuinely cared for his patients. It is worth noting that on this first meeting, Dr Perrin did not promise a 'cure' but a high likelihood of improvement and the possibility of becoming symptom free. He explained that this happens in some, but not all cases.

When it came to Dr Perrin's physical examination of me, I was slightly worried that he may say that I didn't in fact have ME/CFS. He said that not every patient presenting in his clinic has ME/CFS.

In some way I was relieved to hear that I actually did have the 'diagnostic' symptoms of ME/CFS, and that I wasn't just 'lazy or crazy'. On the other hand, I suspected that there was a hard road ahead before I had any improvement.

With the encouragement of my girlfriend Cathy, I decided to commit to six months of the Perrin treatment to see what could be done. Unfortunately a 'miracle' did not happen.

I was told by Dr Perrin not to expect 'miracles' and that a long-term illness (twenty plus years) will require a long term strategy, to move towards recovery. Within the first month I started to feel worse. I was told that this was a possibility and, in some ways, a positive sign. Dr Perrin said that the toxins clearing through my body could cause this effect.

After a number of months of treatment, I started to notice improvements. I was feeling more relaxed and rested in the evenings, friends and family mentioned that I seemed to be more energetic and had a better colour, and an improved mood.

The treatment progress was slow and unsteady, with some days better than others, but improvement persisted.

Thanks to the encouragement and support from my girlfriend Cathy, this improvement has continued with good days and bad days, but consistently improving season on season.

I have had a good number of years of the Perrin treatment to get to this point. In the beginning weekly and then fortnightly and now rarely, and I have done the self-massage treatments at home daily. I knew that my very best chance of becoming symptom free from ME/CFS was by following Dr Perrin's protocol to the letter.

I had heard that there was only a 17 percent chance of becoming fully symptom free with 'The Perrin Technique', but I used to say to Cathy "Who does absolutely everything to the letter? The odds of getting better in my opinion are more like 50/50"

I was determined to get better and I would not stop until I achieved that goal. It took some time to fully listen to my body instead of 'pushing through' and I combined the Perrin treatments with rest, a healthy diet, daily meditation and Chi Gung/Tai Chi practise.

If I could have this time over, I would take the fifty per cent rule of Dr Perrin's more seriously from the very beginning. I would stringently only do half of what I felt I could do with every task. Failing to adhere to this set back my recovery at times. Now I follow this rule, it has been an integral part in allowing me to rest and recuperate.

The improvements have been significant and reading back through my own life story it is hard to recognise the person that I was before I started treatment with Dr Perrin. The speed of progress has been slow and gradual, but the distance covered has made the whole journey worthwhile.

It is hard to put into words just how grateful I am to Dr Perrin, for all he has done for me. His insight, his wisdom, his talent for healing, and his sense of fun and laughter has helped get me through. No matter how ill I felt turning up to the clinic, I always knew I could rely on Dr Perrin to make me feel better. Thank you for putting me on the 'path to healing'.

'The Perrin Technique' has changed my life so much for the better, as it has other ME/CFS sufferers whom I know, that I then qualified as a 'Perrin Technique Practitioner' under Dr Raymond Perrin and I worked with him at The Perrin Clinic, in Prestwich.

Since working with Dr Perrin, I started treating ME and fibromyalgia patients and now Long Covid patients at the Fulwood Therapy Centre.

I now work one-on-one with ME/CFS patients, and my struggles and challenges on my journey inform my ability to guide and support my patients through to improved health.

I continue to research various natural healing modalities to continue to improve my health, and to help my patients to do the same.

Mark Singleton - The Author Cathy's Partner and son of James Singleton (Former Head of Clinical Psychology at RPH), 'The Perrin Technique Practioner' at The Fulwood Therapy Centre, on Black Bull Lane, Fulwood, Preston, Lancashire.

Contact Perrin Practitioner Mark Singleton: *www.marksingleton.me*

In the middle of May, I step out into the heavily wooded forest, surrounded by trees bowing in the breeze, observing an ever dimming yellow-orange sunset ahead in the distance. I am filled with inner peace and serenity.

With a natural complexion and a relaxed stance, I tip toe gently through the soft green bladed grass under exposed bare feet, and I smile at how beautiful the painted picturesque scene surrounds are, and marvel at just how far I have come. I stand beside a large flaked brown oak tree, and extend both arms, embracing the tree in gratitude.

In meditation, I offer thanks at how lucky I am to be alive, and to able to walk again. Looking through a portal of trees, I encourage the energy within the forest to align with my own inner healing energy. Within this practised meditative state, I am once more rejuvenated and filled with increased oxygen and enlightenment, from the beauty of nature's surrounds.

Happy and peaceful in my own company, and no longer needing an applause myself, I inwardly applaud and thank all the people whom I have been blessed to know on my healing journey. All the love and support and new friendships I have received along the way, filled with such warmth and generosity of the human spirit. I feel honoured to know these people.

My future is unknown, but my dreams are filled with gratitude, hope and passion. I have a new found purpose to help and serve others through multiple modalities, so that my journey will not be in vain, and so that my story may never be repeated. I am joyful, peaceful and healthy, and I wish the reader the same in abundance…

I hope that the reader has enjoyed reading my story, and I leave you with my disclaimer, from an ethereal character I once played in my childhood:

A Midsummer Night's Dream by William Shakespeare. Act V scene 1.

Puck:
"If we shadows have offended,
Think but this, and all is mended,
That you have but slumbered here
While these visions did appear.
And this weak and idle theme,
No more yielding but a dream,
Gentles, do not reprehend:
if you pardon, we will mend:
And, as I am an honest Puck,
If we have unearned luck
Now to escape the serpent's tongue,
We will make amends ere long:
Else the Puck a liar call;
So, good night unto you all.
Give me your hands, if we be friends,
And Robin shall restore amends."

I would like to conclude my book in the words of my dear friend Richard Shillington who has helped support me throughout my healing journey. Shilly always brought copious amounts of humour ensuring me that "It will be all right in the end… and if it's not alright, it's not the end!"

> *I first met Crazy Cathy in 2006 when she was giving drama and acting sessions to children of all ages, including my six-year-old niece Willow.*
> *I couldn't believe how much energy this dynamo had. 10lbs of crazy in a 5lb bag!*
> *She gave 100 percent all of the time and the kids gave it back, not because they had to but because they wanted to and enjoyed it so much.*
> *Cathy has helped so many children with self-confidence and self-worth who have gone on to become better versions of themselves because of the time she spent passing on her knowledge, and passion for theatre and comedy.*
> *Her strength of character, as well as her spirit is extraordinary. Everything that has knocked her down has made her stronger, wiser and more determined than ever. I am not only happy but honoured and humble to call her a true friend.*
> *My name is Richard Shillington. I am a disabled, three-time decorated war veteran, and I believe that Cathy has the heart of strength and soul that any of my brothers in arms have had.*
> **L/Cpl R Shillington (Retd) - 14/20 King's Hussars, and King's Royal Hussars 1987-2001.**

"Friendship isn't a big thing, it's a million little things." - Paulo Coelho.

Thank you to everyone both inside and outside of my book for your kind hearts, invaluable support and wonderful friendships. My life has been more positively enriched by having you in it. I am truly blessed to know you all.

A final special thank you to my publisher Robert Oulds at The Bruges Group for believing in me and having the same passion and desire for helping others, and thus enabling this book to reach as many people as possible in order to help save lives. Thank you also to Mark Crook who brought the light into my world, thus connecting me to my publisher and encouraging me to share 'The Truth About ME'.

The future of ME - 'All truth passes through three stages. First, it is ridiculed. Second, it is violently opposed. Third, it is accepted as being self-evident.
Arthur Schopenhauer - German Philosopher.

Contact Catherine Vandome on *www.catherinevandome.com* or *via social media platforms.*

Endorsements
The future of ME

'All truth passes through three stages. First, it is ridiculed. Second, it is violently opposed. Third, it is accepted as being self-evident.'
Arthur Schopenhauer - German Philosopher

"I first met Miss Cathy Vandome in June 2017. At that time she was housebound owing to the severity of her ME symptoms. Cathy had previously been a highly active entertainer and stand-up comedian, and she was struggling to come to terms with the debilitating effects of her condition.
I have always been impressed by Cathy's determination to recover. She has been in regular contact with me over the years and I have assisted her with her campaign to have ME recognised through as a physical and not a psychological condition.
     "Cathy introduced me to Dr Raymond Perrin who has been instrumental in her recovery process. Cathy is keen to see Dr Perrin's treatment included in the NICE guidelines as a recommended treatment for ME, so that other patients can be supported in this way. Cathy is an enthusiastic and relentless campaigner, despite her physical limitations. I wish her every success with her recovery and her mission to help others"
The Rt Hon Sir Ben Wallace - Secretary of State for Defence and head of the Ministry of Defence (2019 - 2023) Conservative MP for Wyre and Preston North (2010 -2024)

"I once heard a fascinating observation from someone who cycled from Land's End to John of Groats in aid of an ME charity. The Charity arranged for him to stay with ME families along his route. As he handed the cheque over, he said "There's one thing about this condition ME that I don't understand. Does it only affect nice people or can it affect anyone and then makes them nice"
Dr Nigel Speight: MA, MB, B Chir, FRCP, FRCPCH, DCH Paediatrician. Durham

"I cannot and nor do I ever claim to 'cure' a physical illness. NLP is about teaching a positive mindset which can alter neurological patterns in the brain, alongside belief systems, which in turn can positively affect choices that we make in life, but I cannot cure a physical illness."
Dr Richard Bandler (credited to Dr Richard Bandler Co - Creator of NLP) - used with the express permission of Dr Richard Bandler.

"Cathy went on to do amazing performances. I remember thinking "I wish I could sing" and Cathy said to me "I could if I tried". I obviously couldn't, but Cathy was always so positive and she made everyone she met feel like Orville and Keith Harris. Every time I said "I can't" Cathy would simply reply "You can!""

Patrick Monahan (Stand-up Comedian - winner of ITV1 Stand-up comedy 'Show me the funny" at the 'London Hammersmith Apollo" in 2011. TV credits include BBC1, BBC2, ITV1, ITV2, CH4, CH5 and Sky. TV shows include 'Splash' 'Celebrity Squares' 'Let's Dance' for Sports Relief. Currently touring National Theatres and Arts Centres across the UK and has performed over sixteen years at the Edinburgh Festival.)

"I performed on stage with Cathy at a number of venues over the two years that followed and was blown away by her ability to never waste a breath, whether it was delivering gags or singing extremely challenging songs in a way that can only be described as 'dynamic'. Cathy is a born performer, energetic, funny and so engaging."

Lester Crabtree (Stand-up Comedian and author of 'Born to Die')

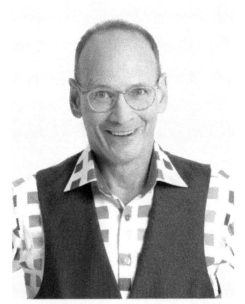

Stand-up Comedian – Steve Royle

"What an amazing story. Catherine's long battle with ME shouldn't be laugh out loud, but somehow it is."

Steve Royle - Stand-up Comedian and finalist of Britain's Got Talent.

THE BRUGES GROUP

The Bruges Group is an independent all-party think tank. Set up in 1989, its founding purpose was to resist the encroachments of the European Union on our democratic self-government. The Bruges Group spearheaded the intellectual battle to win a vote to leave the European Union and against the emergence of a centralised EU state. With personal freedom at its core, its formation was inspired by the speech of Margaret Thatcher in Bruges in September 1988 where the Prime Minister stated, "We have not successfully rolled back the frontiers of the State in Britain only to see them re-imposed at a European level."

We now face a more insidious and profound challenge to our liberties – the rising tide of intolerance. The Bruges Group challenges false and damaging orthodoxies that suppress debate and incite enmity. It will continue to direct Britain's role in the world, act as a voice for the Union, and promote our historic liberty, democracy, transparency, and rights. It spearheads the resistance to attacks on free speech and provides a voice for those who value our freedoms and way of life.

WHO WE ARE

Founder President:
The Rt Hon. The Baroness Thatcher
of Kesteven LG, OM, FRS

Chairman:
Barry Legg

Director:
Robert Oulds MA, FRSA

Washington D.C. Representative:
John O'Sullivan CBE

Founder Chairman:
Lord Harris of High Cross

Former Chairmen:
Dr Brian Hindley
Dr Martin Holmes
& Professor Kenneth Minogue

Academic Advisory Council:
Professor Tim Congdon
Dr Richard Howarth
Professor Patrick Minford
Andrew Roberts
Martin Howe, KC
John O'Sullivan, CBE

Sponsors and Patrons:
E P Gardner Dryden
Gilling-Smith
Lord Kalms
David Caldow
Andrew Cook
Lord Howard
Brian Kingham
Lord Pearson of Rannoch
Eddie Addison
Ian Butler
Thomas Griffin
Lord Young of Graffham
Michael Fisher
Oliver Marriott
Hon. Sir Rocco Forte
Michael Freeman
Richard E.L. Smith

MEETINGS

The Bruges Group holds regular high–profile public meetings, seminars, debates, and conferences. These enable influential speakers to contribute to the European debate. Speakers are selected purely by the contribution they can make to enhance the debate.

For further information about the Bruges Group, to attend our meetings, or join and receive our publications, please see the membership form at the end of this paper. Alternatively, you can visit our website www.brugesgroup.com or contact us at info@brugesgroup.com.

Contact us
For more information about the Bruges Group please contact:
Robert Oulds, Director
The Bruges Group, 246 Linen Hall, 162-168 Regent Street, London W1B 5TB
Tel: +44 (0)20 7287 4414 Email: info@brugesgroup.com

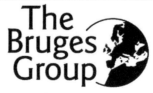

www.brugesgroup.com

Milton Keynes UK
Ingram Content Group UK Ltd.
UKHW030149051224
452010UK00010B/591

9 781739 092085